PROFESSIONAL PARAMEDIC

FOUNDATIONS OF PARAMEDIC CARE

STUDY GUIDE

VOLUME I

MIKE KENNAMER

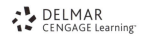

DELMAR
CENGAGE Learning™

Australia • Brazil • Japan • Korea • Mexico • Singapore • Spain • United Kingdom • United States

DELMAR
CENGAGE Learning™

Professional Paramedic: Foundations of Paramedic Care Study Guide
Mike Kennamer

Vice President, Career and Professional
   Editorial: Dave Garza

Director of Learning Solutions: Sandy Clark

Product Development Manager:
   Janet Maker

Managing Editor: Larry Main

Senior Product Manager: Jennifer A. Starr

Editorial Assistant: Amy Wetsel

Vice President, Career and Professional
   Marketing: Jennifer Baker

Executive Marketing Manager:
   Deborah S. Yarnell

Senior Marketing Manager: Erin Coffin

Marketing Coordinator: Shanna Gibbs

Production Director: Wendy Troeger

Production Manager: Mark Bernard

Senior Content Project Manager:
   Jennifer Hanley

Art Director: Benj Gleeksman

ISBN-13: 978-1-4283-2346-9
ISBN-10: 1-4283-2346-5

Delmar
5 Maxwell Drive
Clifton Park, NY 12065-2919
USA

Cengage Learning is a leading provider of customized learning solutions with office locations around the globe, including Singapore, the United Kingdom, Australia, Mexico, Brazil, and Japan. Locate your local office at: **international.cengage.com/region.**

Cengage Learning products are represented in Canada by Nelson Education, Ltd.

To learn more about Delmar, visit **www.cengage.com/delmar.**

Purchase any of our products at your local college store or at our preferred online store **www.cengagebrain.com.**

NOTICE TO THE READER

Publisher does not warrant or guarantee any of the products described herein or perform any independent analysis in connection with any of the product information contained herein. Publisher does not assume, and expressly disclaims, any obligation to obtain and include information other than that provided to it by the manufacturer. The reader is expressly warned to consider and adopt all safety precautions that might be indicated by the activities described herein and to avoid all potential hazards. By following the instructions contained herein, the reader willingly assumes all risks in connection with such instructions. The publisher makes no representations or warranties of any kind, including but not limited to, the warranties of fitness for particular purpose or merchantability, nor are any such representations implied with respect to the material set forth herein, and the publisher takes no responsibility with respect to such material. The publisher shall not be liable for any special, consequential, or exemplary damages resulting, in whole or part, from the readers' use of, or reliance upon, this material.

Printed in the United States of America
1 2 3 4 5 XX 12 11 10

CONTENTS

PREFACE

We are pleased to offer a *Study Guide to accompany Professional Paramedic, Volume I: Foundations of Paramedic Care*. Inside these pages you will find tools to help you practice and prepare for success in your Paramedic program, on the certification exam, and beyond.

Features

This Study Guide contains the following features.

Section I: Case Studies & Practice Questions

Divided by chapters, these features review the terms and concepts that are discussed in the corresponding chapter in the book.

- *Case studies* present a scenario intended to reinforce content contained within each chapter. Each of the case studies highlights a "Decision Time" when you must answer questions on how to treat the patient and a "In Retrospect" when you must reflect on whether or not your decision resulted in a positive outcome. These activities help you develop and fine-tune the decision-making skills that ultimately relate to your success in treating patients.
- *25 to 30 practice questions* per chapter allow you to practice your knowledge of the content presented in *Professional Paramedic, Volume I: Foundations of Paramedic Care*. Questions include a variety of styles—multiple choice, short answer, fill in the blank, and matching—to ensure that you master the content.

Section II: NREMT Skills for Paramedic Certification

This section contains the Paramedic skills that you will be tested on as part of the National Registry exam. You will want to practice the steps in the skills and ensure that you are confident in a successful completion of each skill prior to the exam.

Visit **http://www.nremt.org** for up-to-date information on the National Registry and certification exams.

Section III: Answers to Questions

The answers to the questions provided in this Study Guide offer you an opportunity to evaluate your knowledge of the terms and concepts presented in *Professional Paramedic, Volume I: Foundations of Paramedic Care*.

About the Technical Writer: Mike Kennamer, EdD, EMT-P

Mike Kennamer serves as Director of Workforce Development at Northeast Alabama Community College, where he previously served as EMS Program Director and Division Chair. Dr. Kennamer is author of *Basic Infection Control for Health Care Providers* and *Math for Health Care Professionals*, both published by Delmar Cengage Learning. He has also contributed to a number of other Delmar projects.

About the Authors of the Series

Richard Beebe, MS, BSN, NREMT-P

Richard Beebe is the program director for Bassett Healthcare's Center for Rural Emergency Medical Services Education in Cooperstown, New York; a Clinical Assistant Professor at the State University of New York at Cobleskill, New York; and a practicing field paramedic with the Guilderland Police Department.

Dr. Jeff Myers, DO, EdM, NREMT-P, FAAEM

Dr. Myers is board certified in Emergency Medicine. He is currently on faculty at the State University of New York, University at Buffalo; and he serves as the Associate System EMS Medical Director and EMS Fellowship Director at the Erie County

Medical Center, where he is an active member of the physician response team. Dr. Myers is also the assistant medical director for Rural Metro Medical Services of Western New York, based out of Buffalo, New York.

Also Available

- *Professional Paramedic, Volume II: Medical Emergencies, Maternal Health, and Pediatrics*/Order#:978-1-4283-2351-3
- *Study Guide to accompany Professional Paramedic, Volume II: Medical Emergencies, Maternal Health, and Pediatrics*/Order#:978-1-4283-2352-0
- *Professional Paramedic, Volume III: Trauma Care and EMS Operations*/Order#:978-1-4283-2348-3
- *Study Guide to accompany Professional Paramedic, Volume III: Trauma Care and EMS Operations*/Order#:978-1-4283-2349-0

Please visit us at our *Online Companion* site for more learning tools for the Professional Paramedic series, as well as to view other EMS titles: **http://www.cengage.com/community/ems**

ACING THE CERTIFICATION EXAM: AN INTRODUCTION TO TEST-TAKING STRATEGIES

Introduction

Test time. Whether you are preparing for a certification test or a hiring test, the thought of an examination strikes fear in many people's hearts. The fear is so common that psychologists even have a diagnosis called test anxiety. However, testing does not have to be that way. Evaluations are simply an instrument to determine if you were effectively taught the information intended, or if you have the knowledge base necessary to do the job. That's all! If the purpose of testing is so simple, then why do so many people become so anxious when test time comes? Several factors play into test anxiety and why so many people have such fears of testing. However, these can be overcome. With the assistance of this guide, you too can be better prepared and calmer on examination day.

Test Obstacles

Test obstacles are issues that complicate test taking. If we view test taking as simply an avenue to determine the individual's comprehension of the material, then test obstacles are barriers to the process. There are many issues that may create test obstacles. We will discuss a few.

Mental

Mental test obstacles can sometimes be the greatest hurdles to overcome. Mental preparation for a test can be as important as intellectual preparation. So often, many people have failed an exam before they even begin. Issues that arise out of mental obstacles are:

- feeling unprepared
- feeling incompetent
- fear of taking tests
- fear of failure

Overcoming these obstacles can be your greatest asset when testing. Not allowing yourself to be beaten before entering the testing area can make the difference between success and failure on the exam.

Physical

Improper rest, poor eating habits, and lack of exercise can be some of the physical obstacles to overcome. When preparing for tests, always ensure that you get plenty of rest the night before, have a well-balanced meal before the test, and ensure you have a regiment of proper exercise. Physical obstacles are typically the easiest to overcome; however, they are the most overlooked.

Emotional

The emotional obstacles are often the most vague with which to deal. Much like mental obstacles, emotional obstacles can cause a person to do poorly on an exam well before they enter the room. Stress related issues that can interfere with test taking are:

- family concerns
- work-related concerns
- financial concerns

Emotional issues can cause a person to lose focus, cloud decision-making skills, and become distracted. Overcoming these obstacles requires a conscious effort to ensure that emotions do not interfere with the test.

Preparing to Take a Test

Before the Test

1. Start preparing for the examination. For certification exams, start the first day of class. You can do this by reading your syllabus carefully to find out when your exams will be, how many there will be, and how much they are weighed into your grade.
2. For certification classes, plan reviews as part of your regular weekly study schedule; a significant amount of time should be used to review the entire material for the class.
3. Reviews are much more than reading and reviewing class assignments. You need to read over your class notes and ask yourself questions on the material you don't know well. (If your notes are relatively complete and well organized, you may find that very little rereading of the textbook for detail is needed.) You may want to create a study group for these reviews to reinforce your learning.
4. Review for several short periods rather than one long period. You will find that you are able to retain information better and get less fatigued.
5. Turn the main points of each topic or heading into questions and check to see if the answers come to you quickly and correctly. Do not try to guess the types of questions; instead, concentrate on understanding the material.

During the Test

1. Preview the test before you answer anything. This gets you thinking about the material. Make sure to note the point value of each question. This will give you some ideas on how best to allocate your time.
2. Quickly calculate how much time you should allow for each question. A general rule of thumb is that you should be able to answer 50 questions per hour. This averages out to one question every 1.2 seconds. However, make sure you clearly understand the amount of time you have to complete the test.
3. Read the directions CAREFULLY. (Can more than one answer be correct? Are you penalized for guessing?) Never assume that you know what the directions say.
4. Answer the easy questions first. This will give you confidence and a feel for the flow of the test. Only answer the ones for which you are sure of the correct answer.
5. Go back to the difficult questions. The questions you have answered so far may provide some indication of the answers.
6. Answer all questions (unless you are penalized for wrong answers).
7. Generally, once the test begins, the proctor can ONLY reread the question. He/she cannot provide any further information.
8. Circle key words in difficult questions. This will force you to focus on the central point.
9. Narrow your options on the question to two answers. Many times, a question will be worded with two answers that are obviously inaccurate, and two answers that are close. However, only one is correct. If you can narrow your options to two, guessing may be easier. For example, if you have four options on a question, then you have a 25% chance of getting the question correct when guessing. If you can narrow the options to two answers, then you increase to a 50% chance of selecting the correct choice.
10. Use all of the time allotted for the test. If you have extra time, review your answers for accuracy. However, be careful of making changes on questions of which you are not sure. People often change the answers to questions of which they were not sure, when their first guess was correct.

After the Test

Relax. The test has been turned in. You can spend hours second-guessing what you could have done, but the test is complete. For certification tests, follow up to see if you can find out what objectives you did well and what areas you could improve. Review your test if you can; otherwise, try to remap the areas of question and refocus your studying.

Summary

Test taking does not have to be overwhelming. The obstacles to testing can be overcome and conquered through solid strategies and preparation. Initiating an effective plan, following it, and mentally preparing for a test can be your greatest tools to test success.

CASE STUDIES & PRACTICE QUESTIONS

CHAPTER **1**

ROLES AND RESPONSIBILITIES OF THE PROFESSIONAL PARAMEDIC

Case Study #1

While enrolled in Paramedic education, you decide to take a public speaking class that will help you to earn your associate's degree. Your first assignment is to prepare a speech about why you chose your current career path.

1. Write the opening paragraph of the speech, explaining why you chose to study paramedicine.

_____

_____

Case Study #2

The day for your first clinical rotation has finally arrived! Today you begin to apply what you have learned in class and labs to real-life experiences. Your first shift is not terribly busy, and you have the good fortune to be able to eat lunch in the hospital cafeteria with Dr. Abel Houston—a veteran emergency physician and your Paramedic program's medical director. The conversation during lunch turns to the practice of paramedicine and how you will be operating under Dr. Houston's medical license. Known as an ardent supporter of paramedicine, Dr. Houston asks you a series of questions intended to make you think about the importance of professionalism. Answer each question in your own words.

1. Why is it important for you to realize that Paramedics operate under the medical license of a physician?

_____

_____

2. What traits set paramedicine apart as a profession?

_____

_____

3. Explain the concept of stewardship in terms of the Paramedic's responsibility to the physician.

_____

_____

4. Why should Dr. Houston, who spent more than a decade studying to earn his medical license, allow you to function under that license?

_____

_____

Practice Questions

Multiple Choice

Select the best answer for each of the following questions.

1. Which of the following is NOT a correct statement?
   a. Paramedicine is an applied science.
   b. The practice of paramedicine is constantly evolving.
   c. Paramedicine is positioned at the intersection of health care, public safety, and public health.
   d. The Paramedic's professional identity is secondary to other roles in which he may serve.

2. Which of the following terms describes the ability to understand what it is like to walk in another person's shoes and develop an emotional understanding of the patient's feelings?
   a. support
   b. sympathy
   c. empathy
   d. emotional vulnerability

3. Which of the following is NOT a *primary* role of the Paramedic?
   a. teacher
   b. patient advocate
   c. clinician
   d. healer

4. Which of the following is the highest level of out-of-hospital provider?
   a. registered nurse
   b. Paramedic
   c. nurse midwife
   d. family practice physician

5. Which of the following describes a Paramedic's scope of practice?
   a. medical practice act
   b. U.S. D.O.T. curriculum
   c. medical control
   d. roles and responsibilities

Short Answer

Write a brief answer to each of the following questions.

6. Why are Paramedics leaders?

   _____

   _____

7. Describe how Paramedic education has changed over the years.

   _____

   _____

8. List at least five of the eight qualities common in all professions.

   _____

   _____

9. How would a national exam for Paramedics help Paramedics to transfer from one geographical area to another?

   _____

   _____

10. What national organization currently provides a certification of practical testing and written examinations for the certification of Paramedics?

_____

_____

11. What national organization speaks on behalf of Paramedics?

_____

_____

12. What did the landmark National Institute of Medicine Reports entitled "EMS at the Crossroads" and "Hospital Based Emergency Care: At the Breaking Point" speak of?

_____

_____

13. What does the mnemonic PEARLS stand for?

_____

_____

14. Compare and contrast sympathy and empathy.

_____

_____

Fill in the Blank

Complete each sentence by adding the appropriate word in the provided blanks.

15. Paramedics are expected to keep abreast of new developments in the field of medicine through involvement in _____ _____.

16. Physicians are authorized to practice medicine in most states through legislation called a _____ _____ _____.

17. Since Paramedics work under the physician's license, paramedicine is a _____ _____ with physicians.

18. By acting under the physician's license, the Paramedic acts in the role of a _____.

19. A superior EMS system is always in a process of review and re-engineering through _____ _____ _____.

20. The practice of leadership depends upon the practice of _____.

21. Although this was not always the case, changes in EMS are now driven by _____.

22. The culmination of Paramedic education should be _____.

23. A nonjudgmental attitude toward the patient, regardless of the personal circumstances, is referred to as _____.

24. When a Paramedic listens and seeks to understand the patient and the patient's concern, regardless of the severity of the problem, she is practicing the process of _____.

25. A set of professional boundaries that apply to a profession may be called a _____ of _____.

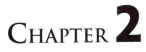

INTRODUCTION TO EMERGENCY MEDICAL SERVICE SYSTEMS

Case Study

Your EMS agency is deeply involved in EMS education and injury prevention in your community. Your supervisor calls you to her office one afternoon to ask you to present a brief history of EMS to an allied health organization at a local high school. You have one week to prepare, and will have one hour to present.

Decision Time

1. Where will you locate reference material with which to prepare your presentation?

   _____

   _____

2. At what point in history will your presentation begin?

   _____

   _____

Considering that you have never done a presentation like this before, you decide to visit your Paramedic instructor to get his input on what you should—and should not—include in your talk. Your instructor is eager to help, and suggests that you watch the pilot episode of *Emergency!*, the television show that inspired him to become a Paramedic. He also recommends that you speak to Dr. Layne, a retired physician who was instrumental in establishing an EMS system in your area.

3. What was the *Emergency!* television show about?

   _____

   _____

4. Make a list of questions that you would ask Dr. Layne.

   _____

   _____

Your presentation is well received, and many students express an interest in becoming a Paramedic. You hope that you will be asked to make similar presentations in the future.

In Retrospect . . .

5. How did you first learn about the EMS profession?

_____

_____

6. What could you learn about the EMS system in your area from experienced Paramedics and physicians?

_____

_____

Practice Questions

Multiple Choice

Select the best answer for each of the following questions.

1. Which of the following events occurred in Roanoke, Virginia, in 1921?
   a. The first ambulance company was established in the United States.
   b. The first fire company was established in the United States.
   c. The first rescue squad was established in the United States.
   d. The first hospital emergency room was established in the United States.

2. When was the first hospital-based ambulance service established in the United States?
   a. 1865
   b. 1869
   c. 1891
   d. 1921

3. How did Dr. Peter Safar demonstrate the safety and efficiency of mouth-to-mouth ventilation in 1958?
   a. with the first "resusci-annie" manikin
   b. by practicing feline intubation
   c. by practicing on anesthetized medical residents
   d. using cadavers

4. Who developed transthoracic defibrillation?
   a. Dr. Barnard Lown
   b. Dr. Paul M. Zoll
   c. Asmund S. Laerdal
   d. Dr. Peter Safar

5. Captain James Page of the Los Angeles Fire Department served as technical advisor for what television show that inspired many to become Paramedics?
   a. *Rescue 9-1-1*
   b. *Adam 12*
   c. *Squad 51*
   d. *Emergency!*

6. Which of the following defines the entire universe of disorders, diseases, syndromes, and skills that an EMS provider might encounter and for which he would be expected to provide emergency care?
   a. National EMS Education Agenda for the Future
   b. National EMS Core Content
   c. National EMS Scope of Practice
   d. National Registry of EMTs

7. Which of the following provides for standardization of EMS providers at all levels?
   a. National EMS Education Agenda for the Future
   b. National EMS Core Content
   c. National EMS Scope of Practice
   d. National Registry of EMTs

8. What is the major advantage of EMS education program accreditation?
   a. gives EMTs the right to practice in each state
   b. serves as the basis for EMS instruction
   c. provides direction for EMS educators
   d. assures the public that graduates will be competent providers

9. Which of the following is NOT represented by a point in the star of life?
   a. detection
   b. reporting
   c. response
   d. definitive care

10. What monumental event took place in Haleyville, Alabama, in 1967?
    a. the first successful resuscitation
    b. the first successful resuscitation using an AED
    c. the first fire-based EMS response
    d. the first 9-1-1 call

11. Which of the following EMS system configurations is dominant in the United States?
    a. fire-based
    b. hospital-based
    c. community-based
    d. municipal

12. Which of the following EMS system configurations was established by groups of physicians and is more common in urban areas?
    a. fire-based
    b. hospital-based
    c. community-based
    d. municipal

13. Which of the following EMS system configurations sometimes results in cross-training among EMS, fire, and law enforcement?
    a. fire-based
    b. hospital-based
    c. community-based
    d. municipal

14. Which of the following EMS system configurations is pressured by a lack of volunteers?
    a. commercial
    b. hospital-based
    c. community-based
    d. municipal

15. Which of the following has placed conditions upon all healthcare providers that protect patient privacy during claims processing, data analysis, utilization review, quality assurance, and practice management?
    a. Health Insurance Portability and Accountability Act
    b. Medical Practice Act
    c. ICD-9
    d. Current Procedural Terminology

Short Answer

Write a brief answer to each of the following questions.

16. When did EMS become recognized as part of the public health services?

_____

_____

17. What is the purpose of the National EMS Core Content?

_____

_____

18. How many levels of EMS providers are delineated by the National EMS Scope of Practice?

_____

_____

19. What is the purpose of a state-issued license?

_____

_____

20. When does certification take place in EMS?

_____

_____

Fill in the Blank

Complete each sentence by adding the appropriate word in the provided blanks.

21. Traditionally EMS was stationed in standing facilities and many EMS services still use the _____-_____ method of resource distribution.

22. System status management (SSM) is an example of _____ _____ deployment.

23. Paramedics called to transport sick and injured patients from outlying clinics and critical access hospitals to tertiary care centers and perform critical care interfacility transportation are involved in the subspecialty called _____ _____ _____.

24. Often retrospective and remedial in nature, _____ _____ is present whenever a physician is involved in quality improvement and provides direction to Paramedics.

25. Medical _____ implies direct involvement in patient care, including on-line medical control.

26. The physician's authority is often exerted through a written set of instructions, called _____.

27. Standing orders are often given to Paramedics in the form of a flowchart format called a/an _____.

Matching

Match each term with its corresponding description.

_____ 28. health maintenance organization

_____ 29. preferred provider organization

_____ 30. point of service

a. a modified fee-for-service schedule that permits patients to choose their healthcare provider from among a roster

b. system that allows a patient to choose a healthcare provider from a list of preferred care providers, although the patient may elect to see another provider for a higher fee

c. system that provides payments to healthcare providers at a negotiated annual per capita rate

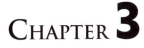

CHAPTER **3**

WORKFORCE SAFETY AND WELLNESS

Case Study #1

As a Paramedic in a small, rural EMS system, you are sometimes called to respond from home to emergencies in your neighborhood, even when you are off duty. On this typical springtime Sunday afternoon you spent most of the day with family enjoying the outdoors. The serenity of the day is interrupted when your pager is activated. A motor vehicle collision has resulted in three serious injuries. The EMS unit from your local station is on the scene, but needs help in dealing with three critical patients. As you start for your car, several things are running through your mind: What route should you take? Should you wear what you have on (shorts and T shirt) or put on a uniform? Is your jump kit in the car?

Decision Time

1. Before taking any action, what is the first thing you should consider?

   _____

   _____

2. Should you take a minute or two to put on a jumpsuit and appropriate shoes or boots, or should you just jump in the car and go?

   _____

   _____

Rather than running directly to the car, you consider the thing that your Paramedic instructor stressed the most—personal safety. Consequently, you take a minute to slip on a jumpsuit—not just because of the uniform identification, but also for the extra protection it provides. You also put on your duty boots and consider the route that you will take as you head for the car.

While en route, you avoid residential streets and drive within the posted speed limit. Although taking preparatory steps and driving the speed limit took a little more time, you know you will arrive safely and prepared for service.

You arrive at the scene to find that a dump truck has hit a coupe head-on. The driver of the dump truck is uninjured, but the occupants of the coupe—three teenage girls—are seriously injured. The driver and front seat passenger have been extricated, and are being attended by the ambulance crew. The senior Paramedic on the scene asks you to treat the back seat passenger, who is being extricated by the fire department. A firefighter/EMT is holding midline axial alignment, and is communicating with the patient during the extrication. You grab a pair of gloves and hastily begin to don them as you hurry to the car. Just as you look in the back window of the car to begin communicating with the EMT, the front seat gives and you find yourself showered with tiny pieces of glass. Uninjured, but embarrassed that you neglected to wear safety glasses, you retreat as you try to shake the wet glass from your clothing and hair.

The patient is extricated and you assist with treatment until she can be transported by a second EMS unit. The driver and passenger were both transported by helicopter, so you help the first responding EMS crew to ready their unit for service.

"Oow! Where did that come from?" asks the senior Paramedic as she focuses on your face for the first time. The blank look on your face lets her know that you are not aware that, along with glass, blood is splattered on your face. "You'd better wash that off," she states, as she directs you to the jump seat in the ambulance.

In Retrospect . . .

While you thought clearly and took adequate safety precautions before you arrived at the scene, the action and severity of the scene contributed to your making a serious mistake of not taking appropriate precautions once on the scene.

3. What type of additional safety precautions should you have taken before approaching the patient?

_____

_____

4. Since blood was splattered on your face, what actions should you take at this time?

_____

_____

5. What can you do to prevent this from happening in the future?

_____

_____

Case Study #2

It is Saturday night in the city, and you feel a sense of dread as you are dispatched to what may be the worst apartment complex in the worst part of town for a domestic disturbance. The police are en route, so you plan to stop a few blocks away until you hear that the scene is safe for you to approach. However, the police arrive first and let you know that the suspect left before their arrival, and that you are cleared to proceed to the patient.

You arrive at the scene and proceed to the third floor, where your patient is located. She is stable, but agitated. Her former boyfriend used a key to let himself into her apartment. Her new boyfriend found this less than amusing, but slipped out in the melee that ensued. Her old boyfriend took it somewhat harder, and threw both verbal and physical blows. As you assess the patient, someone in the hall yells that boyfriend number two—Jerry—has returned to the apartment complex looking for boyfriend number one, and is armed with a gun.

Decision Time

1. What is generally the best option when someone at the scene has a deadly weapon? Is this practical in this circumstance?

_____

_____

2. What is the next best option in this situation?

_____

_____

Since the police are in the apartment with you, they direct you to stay where you are as one law enforcement officer guards the door and other officers search the complex for the suspect. To assure the best cover, you relocate to a room near the center of the apartment, with no windows, no outside access, and several walls between you and the front door.

In Retrospect . . .

The police take the suspect into custody, and though the patient refuses transport, you wait until law enforcement clears you to leave the apartment.

3. How could the outcome of this call have been different if you had not waited for law enforcement to arrive and secure the scene before entering?

_____

_____

4. Although this call took place in a dangerous part of town, a similar scenario could unfold in the best suburban neighborhood as well. How can you help to assure that you do not get caught in the middle of an altercation?

_____

_____

Practice Questions
Multiple Choice

Select the best answer for each of the following questions.

1. Which of the following is defined as the active process of becoming aware of, and making choices toward, a more successful existence?
   a. safety
   b. eustress
   c. wellness
   d. illness

2. You suspect that a coworker is struggling with alcoholism. Alcoholism may be associated with which of the following?
   a. stress
   b. strain
   c. defusing
   d. risk management

3. Which of the following is the correct way to carry an equipment bag?
   a. with the strap over the left shoulder and the bag under the right arm
   b. with the strap at its fullest length
   c. by hand or slung over the shoulder
   d. on the back, like a backpack

4. Which of the following is NOT a good cover object?
   a. fire hydrant
   b. telephone pole
   c. curtain
   d. engine block

5. The Paramedic's health and wellness involves the well-being of all but which of the following aspects?
   a. intellectual
   b. social
   c. spiritual
   d. awareness

6. What percentage of American men are considered to be obese?
   a. 35%
   b. 45%
   c. 50%
   d. 60%

7. Which of the following is considered aerobic exercise?
   a. walking
   b. use of free weights
   c. resistance exercises
   d. strength training

8. Which of the following is associated with the sympathetic nervous system?
   a. catecholamine release
   b. epinephrine release
   c. negative chronotropy
   d. negative inotropy

9. Which of the following is NOT an expected response of stress?
   a. tension headaches
   b. ulcers
   c. muscle relaxation
   d. neck pain

10. Which of the following is NOT a high potential critical incident?
   a. multi-casualty incident
   b. suicide of a family member
   c. line-of-duty death
   d. excessive media exposure

Short Answer

Write a brief answer to each of the following questions.

11. What immunizations are considered standard in most EMS agencies?

   _____

   _____

12. How might a Paramedic protect his patients by keeping up-to-date with personal immunizations?

   _____

   _____

13. Describe body substance isolation.

   _____

   _____

14. Given a choice between cover and concealment in a hazardous situation, which should the Paramedic choose?

   _____

   _____

15. Describe how personal wellness is more than simply the absence of disease.

   _____

   _____

Fill in the Blank

Complete each sentence by adding the appropriate word in the provided blanks.

16. The active process of becoming aware of, and making choices toward, a more successful existence is the definition of _____.

17. A body mass index of 30 or greater indicates _____.

18. Morbid obesity is defined as _____ pounds over ideal weight.

19. The objective of CISD is _____.

20. Post-traumatic stress disorder (PTSD) must be considered if symptoms of acute stress do not resolve within _____ weeks.

21. The leading cause of preventable death is _____.

22. The second leading cause of preventable death is _____.

23. _____ _____ is a plan that emphasizes safety and whose goal is to reduce Paramedic injury in an effort to promote a culture of safety.

24. Safety starts at _____.

25. Paramedics are at the greatest risk of personal injury during the _____ _____ to the scene of an emergency.

26. A defensive driving attitude, or _____ _____ for others on the road, can help to limit the number of motor vehicle collisions.

27. The primary concern of Paramedics upon arrival on the scene of an emergency is _____ _____.

28. Although a safety officer may be charged with the overall responsibility for safety at a large incident, responsibility for overall safety at a small incident falls to the _____-_____-_____.

29. Instruments intended to inflict death and disability are considered _____ _____.

30. An object that, under the right circumstances, could be used to inflict injury or death is considered a _____ _____.

CHAPTER 4

RESEARCH AND EMS

Case Study

As a Paramedic who strives for excellence, you constantly wonder how you can improve patient care. Your interest in improving patient care leads you to consider conducting a research project.

Decision Time

1. What topic will you study? In other words, what question do you want to answer?

   _____

   _____

2. What is your first step?

   _____

   _____

You conduct a literature review to see if the study has already been conducted. Although another Paramedic may not have studied the issue, another healthcare provider may have studied and documented a similar issue.

3. What resources are available for your literature review?

   _____

   _____

4. From whom must you gain approval before conducting research on human subjects?

   _____

   _____

You decide to conduct retrospective research, which allows you to glean information from old patient care reports. Although prospective research is more scientifically valid than retrospective research, there is a place for retrospective research in EMS as well. By partnering in this project with your quality assurance manager and the quality assurance managers at two local hospitals, you are able to expand the breadth of information for which you have access, and add expertise to the research team. Surprisingly, you find that your research question is answered in the negative. In other words, your research hypothesis was proven to be incorrect. Disappointed by your findings, you speak to your medical director to ask what you did wrong. "Nothing," she says. "Research is about finding the answer to our questions. If we already knew all the answers, research would not be needed."

In Retrospect . . .

5. Why is a negative result just as important as an affirmative result?

   _____

   _____

Case Studies & Practice Questions   17

Practice Questions

Multiple Choice

Select the best answer for each of the following questions.

1. Which of the following is the most scientifically valid type of study design?
   a. data dredging
   b. prospective research
   c. retrospective research
   d. literature review

2. Which of the following is the gold standard for research?
   a. prospective research
   b. data mining
   c. double-blinded randomized clinical trial
   d. data analysis

3. What alpha level is considered the standard for probabilities in medical research?
   a. 0.05
   b. 0.50
   c. 0.55
   d. 0.005

4. Which of the following types of research simply states the prevalence of a condition and is often illustrative of a problem, without trying to offer explanation?
   a. case report
   b. descriptive study
   c. observational studies
   d. experimental studies

5. Which of the following types of research asks a question and poses a simple explanation or hypothesis?
   a. case report
   b. descriptive study
   c. observational studies
   d. experimental studies

6. Which of the following types of research starts with a suggested explanation of why something might occur?
   a. case report
   b. descriptive study
   c. observational studies
   d. experimental studies

7. Which type of research error is also called a false positive?
   a. type I error
   b. type II error
   c. type III error
   d. type IV error

8. While conducting your research you find that a patient's blood pressure is elevated, resulting in the patient participating in a diet and exercise program to control the disorder. The blood pressure is later rechecked, revealing a normal reading. However, you later find that the first blood pressure reading was obtained in error, and provided incorrect readings. Which type of research error have you experienced?
   a. type I error
   b. type II error
   c. false negative
   d. null hypothesis

9. Which of the following is an independent ethics committee that is tasked with ensuring that human rights are not violated and the standards of medical research are upheld?
   a. data and safety monitoring board
   b. quality assurance board
   c. Institutional Review Board
   d. safety committee

10. Which of the following is a term borrowed from business that suggests that one method of delivering care is the most effective, and therefore the preferred, means of providing care?
    a. best practice
    b. paradigm blindness
    c. Kaizen
    d. cost-benefit

Short Answer

Write a brief answer to each of the following questions.

11. What is the purpose of scientific EMS research?

    _____

    _____

12. Where did Paramedic practices, protocols, and procedures originate?

    _____

    _____

13. What is a major advantage of evidence-based practice?

    _____

    _____

14. What is the most common type of research found in EMS literature?

    _____

    _____

15. What is the strongest type of research?

    _____

    _____

16. What are the three basic types of research?

    _____

    _____

17. What does the National Research Act of 1974 outline?

    _____

    _____

18. In the absence of research, what can Paramedics use as a way of determining the best method or most effective way of providing patient care?

    _____

    _____

19. What is a type I error in experimental research?

_____

_____

20. What is a type II error in experimental research?

_____

_____

21. How can research help EMS providers to obey Hippocrates' edict to "help or at least to do no harm"?

_____

_____

22. What is the first step to transform a practice to evidence-based practice?

_____

_____

23. What is the advantage of peer-reviewed journals?

_____

_____

Matching

Match each term with its corresponding description.

_____ 24. MEDLINE

_____ 25. PubMed

_____ 26. Educational Resources Information Center (ERIC)

_____ 27. abstract

_____ 28. reference librarian

_____ 29. literature

_____ 30. peer-reviewed

a. circulates submissions to other experts in the field for critical analysis

b. an abbreviated summary

c. most inclusive search engine for medicine

d. search engine of the National Library of Medicine

e. trained in research techniques

f. popular search engine for educational literature research

g. published reports of research

CHAPTER 5

ETHICS AND THE PARAMEDIC

Case Study

As a new Paramedic on a city unit, you are eager to learn all you can about the "real world." Today, you are thrilled to find that you are partnered with Bill Black, a veteran Paramedic of more than 25 years. The day starts with a couple of fairly routine calls—a motor vehicle collision with minor injuries and a fall at a construction site. On your third call—a shortness of breath call in a downtown apartment complex—your partner is rude to the patient's family members. Since you respond to your fourth call with no opportunity for a break, you do not have a chance to speak to Bill about the incident. However, it is on that fourth call of the day that you determine that you must say something.

Your call is to an apartment complex that caters to elderly residents. Your patient is an elderly widow who complains of her heart "fluttering." While you are assessing the patient, your partner asks the patient where to find her medications. She tells him that they are on the kitchen counter. As you continue to assess the patient, you notice that Bill goes to the kitchen to pick up the mediations, but also goes into the patient's bedroom and opens a number of dresser drawers. Since you are busy assessing the patient, you can't see what Bill is doing, but you are uneasy about his wandering around the apartment. Bill finally emerges from the bedroom, and you suggest that he bring in the ambulance cot. Although he knows nothing about the patient assessment you have conducted, he approaches the patient and rudely tells her that Medicare will not pay for her to go to the hospital since it is not medically necessary. When she objects and states that she wants to go to the hospital, Bill becomes even more rude and says "Cash up front, Grandma!"

Decision Time

1. What do you do at this point?

   _____

   _____

You tell your patient that you will take good care of her and that billing matters can be discussed at a later time. You sternly tell Bill to bring in the stretcher, so you can transport the patient to the emergency department. You transport the patient without incident and take care of both the medical and billing paperwork. As you prepare to go back in service before your next call, you wonder if you should discuss the earlier incidents with your partner.

2. Should you take the time to discuss the incidents before you receive another call?

   _____

   _____

3. How will you approach this issue?

   _____

   _____

You decide to speak to Bill about the two issues that concerned you on the previous call, as well as his overt rudeness on an earlier call. His response is that he is "fed up with people who are not sick abusing the system." He further states that "Old people are a drain on the system." You are appalled at his statements and tell him that he needs to keep his opinions to himself and at least act like a professional.

As you complete the rest of an uneventful shift, you consider the following.

In Retrospect . . .

4. Should you report the incident to your supervisor?

_____

_____

5. Should you tell your supervisor about your partner rifling through your patient's dresser drawers?

_____

_____

6. Why do you think that your partner became so jaded that he is rude to patients?

_____

_____

Practice Questions

Multiple Choice

Select the best answer for each of the following questions.

1. What term is used to describe a system of guiding principles that governs a person's conduct?
   a. religion
   b. morals
   c. ethics
   d. conduct

2. Which of the following statements about culture is NOT accurate?
   a. Culture means those unique activities and symbols that make one group's condition different from another.
   b. The prevalent culture in some EMS organizations includes a sense of a higher purpose.
   c. Culture can include special rituals.
   d. EMS has no distinct culture.

3. Which of the following models of ethics states that the end justifies the means?
   a. teleological
   b. utilitarianism
   c. deontological
   d. universal law

4. Which of the following is NOT a central tenet of bioethics?
   a. patient autonomy
   b. human dignity
   c. privacy
   d. judgment

5. Who developed the first medical code of ethics, adopted by the American Medical Association in 1846?
   a. Hippocrates
   b. Socrates
   c. Thomas Percival
   d. Immanual Kant

Fill in the Blank

Complete each sentence by adding the appropriate word in the provided blanks.

6. Ethics is a _____ of guiding principles that govern a person's conduct.

7. Factors that can affect a person's ethics are _____ influences and _____ beliefs.

8. Morality is a Paramedic's personal code of _____.

9. The _____ model of ethics states that the end justifies the means.

10. The deontological approach acknowledges that _____ may occur but that Paramedics must perform their duty.

11. A situation that demands action by any person, as a matter of _____, is called universal law.

12. _____ rights are based on a commonly desired human condition.

13. For an off duty Paramedic to stop at the scene of a serious motor vehicle collision is a _____ obligation.

14. Patient _____ is the patient's ability to control her person and personal destiny through decision making.

15. An adherence to truthfulness is called _____.

Matching

Match each term with its corresponding description.

_____ 16. beneficence

_____ 17. non-maleficence

_____ 18. fidelity

_____ 19. veracity

_____ 20. privacy

_____ 21. patient autonomy

_____ 22. justice

_____ 23. ethical obligation

_____ 24. *primun non nocere*

_____ 25. divine command ethics

a. source of virtues that comes from external sources

b. first, do no harm

c. adherence to truthfulness

d. acts of mercy and charity

e. obligation to keep the promises that are made to the patient

f. no harm will be done

g. secluded from intrusion

h. ability to control one's own destiny

i. application of the concept of fairness

j. responsibility of EMS to respond to calls for help

k. extrinsic source of virtues

CHAPTER 6

THE LAW AND PARAMEDICS

Case Study

Law enforcement calls you to a convenience store where a young man is sitting on a curb in front of a dumpster. As you approach, you see that he has green paint around his nose and mouth, and appears very agitated. The police officer tells you that he and his friends were "huffing" paint when he became groggy and nearly passed out. His friends panicked and called 9-1-1. The police officer says that he does not want to agitate the patient any more than necessary, and prefers that he agree to go to the hospital without being forced to do so. He warns, however, that the patient is very agitated and may have to be arrested, handcuffed, and taken by force.

Decision Time

1. As you approach the patient, what type of consent will you be seeking?

   _____

   _____

2. What will you do if the patient refuses treatment?

   _____

   _____

You make contact with the patient and introduce yourself as a Paramedic. The patient seems to listen to you, but you are uncertain that he is able to comprehend what you are telling him.

3. How can you assure that you have completed all the steps necessary in obtaining informed consent?

   _____

   _____

Your patient decides to cooperate and appears oriented. You explain the benefits of treatment and transport, as well as the alternatives if he does not go to the hospital. You also let him know that he can withdraw consent, the risks involved if he does not seek treatment, and the nature of the procedure. You answer any questions, let him know about his consent rights, inform him of the consequences if he does not accept treatment, and assure yourself that he understands your explanation.

Correctly assuming that he might be going to the hospital with or without his consent, he gives his consent for transport, which takes place without incidence.

In Retrospect . . .

4. How would consent be impacted if the patient was 15 years old?

   _____

   _____

Practice Questions

Multiple Choice

Select the best answer for each of the following questions.

1. Which of the following helps the courts assure fairness under the law?
   a. magistrates
   b. case law
   c. statutes
   d. regulations

2. What authority do the rules and regulations promulgated by government units formed under statutory authority and charged with various functions carry?
   a. the duty to act
   b. the authority of law
   c. the duty of the magistrate
   d. the authority of the king

3. A local industry is fined by the Occupational Safety and Health Administration (OSHA) for unsafe practices in the workplace. What type of judge would hear this type of case?
   a. administrative law judge
   b. appellate court judge
   c. magistrate
   d. circuit court judge

4. Which type of law is involved in a breach of contract case?
   a. criminal law
   b. tort law
   c. administrative law
   d. civil law

5. Which type of law is likely involved in the following case: *State of Alabama v. Jacob Genheim*?
   a. criminal law
   b. tort law
   c. administrative law
   d. civil law

6. Which of the following is NOT a required element of a tort?
   a. duty to act
   b. breach of duty
   c. abandonment
   d. causation

7. Which of the following best describes Good Samaritan legislation in most states?
   a. Off-duty Paramedics have a duty to help the sick and injured.
   b. An unlicensed individual is required to stop to help an injured traveler.
   c. People who stop to help an injured person are immune from lawsuits.
   d. Healthcare providers who have no duty to act are protected from liability.

8. Which of the following terms is used to describe the charge brought when a Paramedic performs the correct procedure, but does so incorrectly?
   a. malfeasance
   b. misfeasance
   c. nonfeasance
   d. disfeasance

9. Which charge could be brought if a Paramedic gives an IV bolus to a hypertensive head-injured patient?
   a. malfeasance
   b. misfeasance
   c. nonfeasance
   d. disfeasance

10. Which charge would be brought if the patient dies as a result of an equipment malfunction that could have been prevented under normal circumstances?
    a. malfeasance
    b. misfeasance
    c. nonfeasance
    d. disfeasance

Short Answer

Write a brief answer to each of the following questions.

11. Explain how you can assure that you have completed all the necessary steps in obtaining informed consent.

   _____

   _____

12. How are advanced directives different from acting against medical advice (AMA)?

   _____

   _____

13. What are the four core principles included within the concept of advanced directives?

   _____

   _____

14. Describe the concept of legitimate interest relative to confidential patient information.

   _____

   _____

15. How does case law help to assure consistent application of the law?

   _____

   _____

Matching

Match each term with its corresponding description.

_____ 16. deposition

_____ 17. subpoena

_____ 18. summary judgment

_____ 19. affidavit

_____ 20. settlement

_____ 21. motion

_____ 22. summary dismissal

_____ 23. statute of limitations

_____ 24. negligence per se

_____ 25. expressed consent

_____ 26. verbal consent

_____ 27. disclosure

_____ 28. age of majority

_____ 29. legal capacity

_____ 30. witness

a. a function of mental state and age

b. patient gives oral approval for treatment

c. legal age in a given state

d. plaintiff cannot commence a lawsuit after a certain time has passed

e. one who can attest

f. the assumption that care is wanted if the patient does not object

g. sworn written statement which attests to facts involving the case

h. request for some action from the judge

i. clear understanding of the implications of treatment

j. legal command to appear in a certain place and time

k. formal proceeding prior to the trial in which a witness answers questions under oath

l. throwing out the case on its lack of merit

m. summary judgment granted to plaintiff

n. agreement to pay a sum of money to conclude a matter outside of court

o. outcome of case decided on court filings

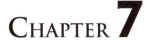
CHAPTER 7

PUBLIC HEALTH AND THE PARAMEDIC

Case Study

You are called to a suburban neighborhood on a reported "sick call." Your patient is a 58-year-old Asian man who stayed home from work today because he felt ill. You arrive to find the patient complaining of flu-like symptoms. His wife tells you that he just returned from a business trip to Indonesia, and that she is afraid he has contracted the swine flu.

Decision Time

1. What precautions will you take as you begin to assess this patient?

_____

_____

You don a mask and gloves and begin to assess the patient. The patient's wife insists that the patient has swine flu because he doesn't wash his hands enough when he is traveling. Although you believe her "diagnosis" to be unlikely, you take all precautions to protect your patient, your crew, and yourself.

2. What health agency should be notified if the physician suspects a reportable communicable disease?

_____

_____

You later learn that the patient is suffering from the common cold, and does not have swine flu.

In Retrospect . . .

3. What would you have done differently if the patient did have swine flu?

_____

_____

Practice Questions

Fill in the Blank

Complete each sentence by adding the appropriate word in the provided blanks.

1. Public health is defined as the practice and discipline of improving the health of _____.

2. The public health team is made up of both _____ _____ and _____.

3. _____ is the branch of medical science that deals with the incidence, distribution, and control of disease in a population.

4. _____ _____ is considered the physical, chemical, biological, and psychosocial well-being of a person as it is related to the natural environment.

5. Social and _____ health addresses issues that are important to the well-being of the population.

6. The field of _____ health is responsible for helping to maintain safety within workplaces.

7. Disaster planning and response begins with the examination of _____ public disasters.

8. The public health movement was first started by public health _____.

9. The partnership between EMS providers and _____ _____ officials is vital to reducing morbidity and mortality in disaster situations.

10. The Occupational Safety and Health Administration is the federal agency responsible for developing and enforcing various standards of safety in the _____.

11. Public health is primarily focused on _____ of illness and injury.

12. A secondary mission of public health is _____ to disease outbreaks and disasters.

13. The practice of _____ can be traced back to biblical times when lepers were forced to live outside the city walls.

14. Outbreaks of diseases that spread throughout a region are considered to be _____.

15. Founded in 1948, the World Health Agency is a specialized health agency under the _____ _____.

16. The Centers for Disease Control and Prevention was founded in 1946 to control _____.

17. The Occupational Safety and Health Administration was founded in 1971 to reduce and prevent _____ -related injuries, illness, and death.

18. For those with no primary care _____, hospital emergency departments serve as a site for preventive medical care.

19. Lillian Wald, RN, was credited with coining the term _____ _____ nurse.

20. The number of agencies that comprise the U.S. Public Health Service is _____.

Matching

Match each term with its corresponding description.

_____ 21. World Health Organization

_____ 22. Surgeon General

_____ 23. Public Health Service

_____ 24. Centers for Disease Control and Prevention

_____ 25. Occupational Safety and Health Administration

a. provides logistical support to public health departments

b. focuses research and policy efforts on emerging infectious diseases

c. monitors disease outbreaks, develops and administers vaccines

d. leads public health service

e. develops and enforces workforce safety standards

CHAPTER **8**

ILLNESS AND INJURY PREVENTION

Case Study

You are called to a loading dock at an abandoned building in the city where a teenage boy has been injured while skateboarding with his friends. You arrive to find that one of the young men has fallen and injured his right arm. You assess him and find that he tried to catch a fall and placed all his weight on his right arm. His wrist is painful, bruised, and swollen. As you assess and treat your patient, you notice that there are a dozen teenage boys who have been "extreme" skateboarding on the rails, stairs, and ramps around the loading dock, but none of them are wearing any protective equipment, such as pads or helmets.

Decision Time

1. Is this a teaching moment for the teenagers?

   _____

   _____

2. How should you approach this issue?

   _____

   _____

As your partner splints the injury, you take time to speak to the other teenagers who are gathered around their friend. You share your concern that they are not protecting themselves with the appropriate personal protective equipment, and that this abandoned factory might not be the safest place to skate. Although you heard much bravado from the boys about how tough they are, you can only hope that your concerns were heard. You take the opportunity to capitalize on another teaching moment while transporting your patient to the hospital. He tells you that the boys hang out at the old factory almost every afternoon. When asked about personal protective equipment, he deflects your concerns by saying, "We don't have helmets and pads, but we make up for it by being tough." When asked about why they chose the old loading dock over one of the nearby skate parks, he replied that he and his friends would not be welcome at those parks. "They make you wear helmets and pads there," he says.

As you leave the hospital to return to the station, you and your partner discuss the situation and wonder if there is something more you can do. "I wonder if they would wear helmets and pads if they had them," your partner says. "And then maybe they would go to skate parks instead of the abandoned factory," you add.

3. Can you see the beginnings of an injury prevention program in this?

   _____

   _____

You and your partner work with a local civic organization to secure the funds necessary to purchase pads and helmets for these skaters. A few days later, you return to the loading dock to find the boys skateboarding on the ramps and rails. As you drive up, the boys stop what they are doing and meet you as you get out of the ambulance with bags of helmets and pads. Although the boys are hesitant to take the gifts at first, they quickly relent and just as quickly start trying on their new equipment. Not forgetting that wearing protective equipment is only one part of the problem, you make sure you invite the boys to a local skateboard park, since they are now "tricked out" with their new equipment. You ask the boys to meet you there the next afternoon.

In Retrospect . . .

The boys meet you at the skate park and show off their tricks as you and your partner watch.

4. What type of equity does this injury program utilize?

   _____

   _____

5. Can this program be expanded to assist others?

   _____

   _____

Practice Questions

Fill in the Blank

Complete each sentence by adding the appropriate word in the provided blanks.

1. Injury and illness _____ is the first step in injury and illness prevention.

2. For public health officials to make good decisions, they need _____ information.

3. Injury statistics are compiled in the National _____ Registry.

4. EMS agencies are community-based organizations that blend public safety with public _____.

5. According to Haddon, if an agent cannot be eliminated, then perhaps it can be reduced to a _____ level.

6. If a hazard cannot be eliminated or reduced, then perhaps it can be _____ to prevent its release or use.

7. In Haddon's countermeasures, the first E is _____.

8. In Haddon's countermeasures, the second E is _____.

9. In Haddon's countermeasures, the third E is law _____.

10. In Haddon's countermeasures, the fourth E is _____ initiatives.

11. The concept of fairness is called _____.

12. The concept of fairness that can be broadly applied to all individuals is called _____ _____.

13. When an injury prevention program benefits a targeted group, it is called _____ _____.

14. When Paramedics capitalize on an opportunity to educate a patient about injury prevention, that opportunity is called a _____ _____.

15. _____ _____ is a matter of comparing the level of injury or illness before and after the program.

Matching

Match each term with its corresponding description.

_____ 16. Ralph Nader

_____ 17. William Haddon, Jr.

_____ 18. National Trauma Registry

_____ 19. National Centers for Injury Prevention and Control

_____ 20. teachable moment

_____ 21. process evaluation

_____ 22. outcomes evaluation

_____ 23. national injury prevention and control centers

_____ 24. Haddon's Countermeasures

_____ 25. Stigma

a. when a patient has a heightened awareness of a problem and is most receptive

b. national network of centers, each with a focus on regional injury interests

c. assesses the efficiency or effectiveness of the injury prevention program's methodology

d. first director of NHTSA

e. early pioneer in public health surveillance

f. assesses the overall effectiveness of the injury prevention program

g. compiles injury statistics submitted by trauma centers

h. engineering, education, enforcement, and economic incentives

i. negative connotation attached to participation in a program

j. created as a result of studies that revealed injury prevention is more cost effective than injury treatment

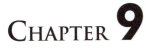

CHAPTER 9

LIFESPAN DEVELOPMENT

Case Study

Your unit is called to the home of a patient who is reportedly complaining of difficulty breathing. When you arrive, you find that the patient is in minor distress. She seems fine, but her daughter is panicky about her mother's condition. Although your partner speaks to the daughter, you learn from the patient that she is terminal, and has been sent home to die. This has greatly upset the patient's daughter.

The patient tells you that her breathing is fine—that she simply had a coughing spell that concerned her daughter. Her daughter wants her to seek additional medical opinions because she believes that the patient's doctor is incompetent. Your knowledge of the Kubler-Ross five stages of dying provides a clue as to what the patient and her daughter are experiencing.

Decision Time

1. What stage of dying is the patient in?

   _____

   _____

2. Clearly, the daughter has not yet reached this stage. What stage is she likely in?

   _____

   _____

3. Should you insist that the patient go to the hospital?

   _____

   _____

Your partner has failed in calming the patient's daughter. They come back in and you wonder if this is a good time for a teaching moment for the daughter.

4. Is it your role to provide grief counseling for this family?

   _____

   _____

In Retrospect . . .

Knowing the five stages of dying will help you to better understand a patient's response to dying, as well as the responses of the patient's family members.

5. What can you do to better use this knowledge to help your patients?

   _____

   _____

Practice Questions

Multiple Choice

Select the best answer for each of the following questions.

1. Which of the following types of development includes bodily changes that are evident throughout life?
   a. personal development
   b. physical development
   c. cognitive development
   d. affective development

2. Which of the following types of development depends upon external societal influences and internal psychological dynamics?
   a. personal development
   b. physical development
   c. cognitive development
   d. affective development

3. Which of the following types of development includes the ability to think and reason?
   a. personal development
   b. physical development
   c. cognitive development
   d. affective development

4. Which of the following is the visible, outward expression of the chromosome?
   a. genotype
   b. gene
   c. phenotype
   d. teratogens

5. Which of the following refers to the division of a cell?
   a. mitosis
   b. blastocyst
   c. embryo
   d. labor

6. Which of the following is NOT a factor in infant mortality?
   a. domestic violence
   b. advanced maternal age
   c. absence of prenatal care
   d. presence of recessive gene

7. A precipitous delivery is one that lasts for how long?
   a. 1 hour or less
   b. 2 to 4 hours
   c. 24 hours or more
   d. 6 to 12 hours

8. During the first minute of life, the umbilical blood flow diminishes. This action does which of the following?
   a. raises O_2 levels
   b. lowers CO_2 levels
   c. stimulates the first breath
   d. all of the above

9. Which of the following parenting types do not establish boundaries or routines?
   a. permissive
   b. authoritative
   c. authoritarian
   d. nonparenting

10. Which of the following types of parents tend to be aggressive with Paramedics?
    a. permissive
    b. authoritative
    c. authoritarian
    d. nonparenting

11. Which of the following types of parents tend to focus on positive behaviors?
    a. permissive
    b. authoritative
    c. authoritarian
    d. nonparenting

12. Which of the following types of parents are most likely to have higher levels of depression?
    a. permissive
    b. authoritative
    c. authoritarian
    d. nonparenting

13. According to Dr. Robert Sternberg, which of the following is NOT an aspect of love?
    a. commitment
    b. friendship
    c. intimacy
    d. passion

14. What percentage of divorced people eventually remarry?
    a. 32
    b. 50
    c. 82
    d. 90

15. What percentage of married adults cannot or do not want to have children?
    a. 5
    b. 10
    c. 20
    d. 52

Matching

Match each term with its corresponding description.

_____ 16. Sigmund Freud

_____ 17. Erik Erikson

_____ 18. B. F. Skinner

_____ 19. Albert Bandura

_____ 20. Ivan Pavlov

_____ 21. Jean Piaget

_____ 22. Joseph Babinski

_____ 23. Ernst Moro

_____ 24. Arnold Gesell

_____ 25. Diana Baumrind

_____ 26. Lawrence Kohlberg

_____ 27. Robert Sternberg

_____ 28. K. Warner Schaie

_____ 29. Elisabeth Kubler-Ross

_____ 30. World Health Organization

a. fanning of toes and extension of great toe caused by stroking lateral soles of feet as a test of lower motor neurons

b. social influences control personal development

c. behaviorism

d. operant conditioning

e. people develop in building block fashion

f. id, ego, and superego

g. social learning theory

h. typology of parenting

i. developmental milestones

j. when startled, infant will extend both arms

k. five stages of dying

l. six stages and three levels of moral development

m. three components of love

n. called obesity a global health epidemic

o. all intellectual abilities decline at about age 68 while significant loss does not occur until age 80

CHAPTER 10

BASIC HUMAN PHYSIOLOGY

Case Study

Your medical director asks you to speak to his Rotary Club about the injury prevention program that you and your partner developed to provide teenagers with personal protective equipment and a safe place to ride their skateboards. As you eat lunch prior to your presentation, you see a banquet room filled with what seems like hundreds, or thousands, of businesspeople. You are right at home at the scene of an emergency and seem to know no fear. However, here in the banquet room of a local restaurant, you are feeling a bit uncomfortable. Your mouth is dry and your heart seems ready to bound from your chest. Although you can't see your face, you have to assume it is pale. You quickly place your index finger to your wrist to see just how fast your heart is beating; it is fast and bounding. You wonder where a heart monitor is when you need it. As these thoughts go through your mind, the club president stands to call the meeting to order.

Decision Time

1. What is causing these symptoms?

   _____

   _____

2. Which division of the autonomic nervous system is dominating here?

   _____

   _____

3. What chemical mediator is causing the symptoms you are experiencing?

   _____

   _____

Your medical director introduces you, and you walk to the podium to begin your presentation. As you stand before the crowd, which is not nearly as big as you earlier thought, you take a couple of deep breaths, thank your medical director for inviting you, and begin to share your story.

In Retrospect . . .

Once you started talking, your nerves calmed and the stress subsided. In fact, by the time the presentation was over, you had begun to enjoy it. As a Paramedic, you just experienced firsthand the way that the human body helps to cope with stress. While you were nervous, your body was prepared for the extra stress level, and it made you sharper.

4. Other than in times of stress, in what other times and conditions does the sympathetic nervous system help to assure that the body maintains adequate blood flow during times of distress?

   _____

   _____

Practice Questions

Fill in the Blank

Complete each sentence by adding the appropriate word in the provided blanks.

1. The first stage of the general adaption syndrome is the _____ stage.

2. The second stage of the general adaption syndrome is the _____ stage.

3. The final stage of the general adaption syndrome is the _____ stage.

4. Daily, ongoing stress is called _____.

5. Neurons are separated by a gap called the _____.

6. Norepinephrine is the chemical mediator for the _____ nervous system.

7. The neurotransmitter of the _____ nervous system is acetylcholine.

8. Beta$_1$ adrenergic receptors are found in abundance in the _____.

9. Found in the gastrointestinal tract, _____ receptors relax smooth muscles.

10. _____ is the increase in weight or functional capacity of a tissue or organ beyond what is normal.

Matching

Match each term with its corresponding description.

_____ 11. milieu

_____ 12. homeostasis

_____ 13. lysosomes

_____ 14. mitochondria

_____ 15. anaerobic metabolism

_____ 16. glycolysis

_____ 17. intracellular water

_____ 18. extracellular water

_____ 19. interstitial fluid

_____ 20. intravascular fluid

_____ 21. hydrostatic pressure

_____ 22. edema

_____ 23. isotonic

_____ 24. hypotonic

_____ 25. hypertonic

_____ 26. third spacing

_____ 27. hyperthermia

_____ 28. hypothermia

_____ 29. pyrexia

_____ 30. endotoxins

a. process of dividing glucose

b. too little heat in the body's core

c. water inside the cell

d. metabolism that does not use oxygen

e. too much heat in the body's core

f. internal equilibrium

g. largest organelle in the cell

h. more water and less salt than the solution on the other side of a semipermeable membrane

i. an environment

j. water outside the cell

k. tiny sacs that contain enzymes which can break down proteins

l. poisons from bacteria

m. fluid built up in tissues

n. fluid found in bloodstream

o. fluid leaks from intravascular space into interstitial space

p. balanced solution

q. created by the force behind water

r. fluid between cells

s. fever

t. less water and more salt than fluid on other side of semipermeable membrane

CHAPTER **11**

PRINCIPLES OF PATHOPHYSIOLOGY

Case Study

You are called to the scene of a fight in the parking lot of a local bar. Law enforcement is on the scene and has it secured. Your patient is a 29-year-old male who has been stabbed in the abdomen. The patient has lost a good deal of blood. His skin is cool, pale, and clammy. His pulse is rapid and thready, and his breathing is slightly labored.

Decision Time

1. What condition is this patient suffering from?

   _____

   _____

2. Is this patient in compensated or decompensated shock?

   _____

   _____

3. What should your treatment include?

   _____

   _____

Due to the patient's condition, you begin transport as you control the bleeding and administer supplemental oxygen. While en route, you start an IV and monitor the patient's condition. The patient's color and his vital signs begin to improve by the time you reach the hospital.

In Retrospect . . .

Although you started the IV en route, some Paramedics would have started the IV on scene.

4. Describe the advantages and disadvantages of starting the IV while en route.

   _____

   _____

5. Physiologically speaking, why did the patient's vital signs improve by the time you reached the hospital?

   _____

   _____

Practice Questions

Multiple Choice

Select the best answer for each of the following questions.

1. Which of the following is a risk factor that cannot be modified?
   a. age
   b. smoking
   c. obesity
   d. alcohol consumption

2. What is the expected outcome of a disease called?
   a. diagnosis
   b. risk factor
   c. prognosis
   d. final outcome

3. What is the branch of medicine that deals with the study of the causes, distribution, and control of disease in populations?
   a. public health medicine
   b. paramedicine
   c. pathophysiology
   d. epidemiology

4. Which of the following terms is synonymous with the death rate?
   a. morbidity
   b. mortality
   c. epidemiology
   d. epidemic

5. What is the name for the volume of red blood cells, expressed as a percentage of red blood cells in the blood?
   a. hemoglobin
   b. hematocrit
   c. anemia
   d. leukocyte count

6. Which of the following is a chemical mediator released from the mast cell that creates a sensation of pain?
   a. leukotrienes
   b. prostaglandins
   c. anaphylatoxins
   d. kallikrein

7. Organs in which of the body systems are the earliest to suffer in shock?
   a. cardiovascular
   b. reproductive
   c. gastrointestinal
   d. circulatory

8. What is a condition in which intravascular fluids leak into the third space, creating total body edema?
   a. disseminated intravascular coagulation
   b. sepsis
   c. liver shock
   d. anasarca

9. Which body system is the first to respond to hypoperfusion?
   a. renal system
   b. cardiovascular system
   c. pulmonary system
   d. integumentary system

10. What mean arterial pressure is required by the brain to maintain adequate perfusion?
    a. 50 to 60 mmHg
    b. 40 to 50 mmHg
    c. 30 to 40 mmHg
    d. 20 to 30 mmHg

Fill in the Blank

Complete each sentence by adding the appropriate word in the provided blanks.

11. The first step in the pathogenesis of hypoxia is called _____.

12. A _____ is any substance capable of causing cell injury or death.

13. Mechanical injury is due to abrupt and sudden physical forces acting upon the body, such as friction, blunt force, or penetrating force, and is referred to as _____.

14. The effect of electrical current passing through the tissue is called _____.

15. Physical damage to the tissues caused by an imbalance between pressures in the environment and those within the body is referred to as _____.

Matching

Match each term with its corresponding description.

_____ 16. hypoxia

_____ 17. disease

_____ 18. recovery

_____ 19. akinetic

_____ 20. pathophysiology

_____ 21. heart failure

_____ 22. clinical death

_____ 23. environmental risk factors

_____ 24. decompensated shock

_____ 25. exacerbation

_____ 26. liquifactive necrosis

_____ 27. nosocomial

_____ 28. biological death

_____ 29. etiology

_____ 30. mortality

a. return to a former functional capacity

b. death

c. the study of the causes of suffering in the human condition

d. acquired in a hospital

e. without motion

f. absence of vital signs

g. a function of one's lifestyle or occupation

h. abnormal change in the function of cells, tissues, or organs

i. cells liquefy upon death

j. the return of symptoms

k. an assumed origin

l. irreversible death

m. an impaired heart that cannot meet the body's demands for perfusion

n. low oxygen concentrations

o. end-stage of a series of cumulative physiologic derangements typically involving one organ system which goes on to affect the entire body

CHAPTER 12

MEDICAL TERMINOLOGY

Case Study

Your regular partner is off for vacation, so you are partnered today with a newly licensed Paramedic. Your first call is a routine transport from a local long-term care facility to the emergency department. As your partner completes his patient care report, he asks for your advice. "How do I know the right mix of medical terminology and simple English to use when writing my report?" he asks. "It seems that it might be easy to get carried away with medical terminology, but I don't want to sound stupid by not using it," he continues.

Decision Time

1. What is your advice to your partner?

_____

_____

Your partner thanks you for your advice and asks when it is appropriate to use medical terminology with a patient.

2. What is your response to this question?

_____

_____

Your partner thanks you again for the advice. "So it is almost like being bilingual," he says. "If you speak English and Spanish, you speak English to your English-speaking friends and Spanish to your Spanish-speaking friends."
   "Exactly!" you say. "You always want to speak the language that is used where you are."

In Retrospect . . .

3. Why not just use a common language (plain English) so that everyone can understand it?

_____

_____

Practice Questions
Short Answer

Write a brief answer to each of the following questions.

1. Why is it important that Paramedics understand medical terminology?

_____

_____

2. How does one read medical terms with prefixes and suffixes?

_____

_____

3. Should you use medical terminology and abbreviations when speaking to a patient?

_____

_____

4. What should you do if you are uncertain of the correct medical term?

_____

_____

5. Why is it sometimes necessary to spell out medical terms?

_____

_____

Matching

Root Words

Match each root word with its corresponding description.

_____ 6. enter/o   a. mouth

_____ 7. hem/o   b. small intestine

_____ 8. thromb/o   c. blood

_____ 9. onc/o   d. kidneys

_____ 10. ile/o   e. cancer

_____ 11. aden/o   f. intestines

_____ 12. oste/o   g. bone

_____ 13. gloss/o   h. gland

_____ 14. ren/o   i. ear

_____ 15. ot/o   j. clot

Prefixes

Match each prefix with its corresponding description.

_____ 16. a/-   a. without

_____ 17. leuko/-   b. white

_____ 18. neo/-   c. below or beneath

_____ 19. levo/-   d. left

_____ 20. homo/-   e. suffering

_____ 21. orth/-   f. beyond or high

_____ 22. phlebo/-   g. same

_____ 23. patho/-   h. straight

_____ 24. hypo/-   i. new

_____ 25. hyper/-   j. vein

Suffixes

Match each suffix with its corresponding description.

_____ 26. -ectasis   a. speech

_____ 27. -algia   b. blood

_____ 28. -phasia   c. inflammation

_____ 29. -itis   d. disease

_____ 30. -iasis   e. swelling

_____ 31. -pathy   f. formation

_____ 32. -edema   g. fear

_____ 33. -emia   h. pain

_____ 34. -phobia   i. expansion

_____ 35. -spasm   j. contraction

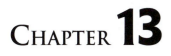

CHAPTER **13**

SCENE SIZE-UP AND PRIMARY ASSESSMENT

Case Study

You are called to an office building where a middle-aged man has collapsed.

Decision Time

1. What is your first priority?

   _____

   _____

Upon arriving, you determine the scene to be safe and proceed to a break room where the patient has collapsed. He does not respond when you walk in the room or when you speak to him. You approach the patient and apply a sternal rub, to which he does not respond.

2. What is the patient's level of consciousness on the AVPU scale?

   _____

   _____

3. What should you do next?

   _____

   _____

4. If the patient is breathing at a rate of eight breaths per minute and shallow, what should you do?

   _____

   _____

You check the patient and find that he has a pulse of 40 beats per minute.

5. Will you continue your assessment on scene or en route?

   _____

   _____

You continue your assessment en route and take the patient to the nearest emergency department. The hospital is nearby, so you do not have time to do much more than support the patient's ventilation and oxygenation and assure an open airway.

In Retrospect . . .

6. Since you didn't have time to start an IV or fully assess the patient, should you have considered delaying transport until this could be done?

_____

_____

Practice Questions

Fill in the Blank

Complete each sentence by adding the appropriate word in the provided blanks.

1. The primary goal of the _____ _____ is to find and manage any of the patient's life-threatening injuries or conditions.

2. _____ priority patients are transported immediately, with further assessment performed en route.

3. Assessment for _____ priority patients is typically conducted in a focused manner while remaining on the scene.

4. Body substance isolation (BSI) creates a _____ between the Paramedic and possibly infectious materials with the use of gloves, masks, gowns, and eye protection.

5. The first step in the initial assessment is to integrate the observations obtained in the scene survey into a _____ _____ of the patient's condition.

6. In the acronym AVPU, the V stands for _____.

7. In the acronym AVPU, the U stands for _____.

8. A patient who is oriented to person, time, and place is considered _____ and _____ times three.

9. A _____ rub is performed by applying the knuckles of one hand on the patient's chest and moving them in a firm, circular motion.

10. Assessing the airway can be simplified to the mantra _____, _____, and _____.

11. If two or more ribs are broken in two or more places, the injury is called _____ _____.

12. Ventilatory support should be considered when the patient's ventilatory rate is less than _____ or greater than _____.

13. The first set of vital signs are considered _____ vital signs.

14. Subsequent sets of vital signs are considered _____ vital signs.

15. A patient who does not respond to a verbal or painful stimulus is said to be _____.

Matching

Match each term with its corresponding description.

_____ 16. airway assessment

_____ 17. scene size-up

_____ 18. initial assessment

_____ 19. mechanism of injury

_____ 20. general impression

_____ 21. body substance isolation

_____ 22. jaw thrust

_____ 23. alert

_____ 24. poor general impression

_____ 25. serial vital signs

a. clue to life-threatening condition

b. event that caused harm to the patient

c. used to illustrate trends in vital sign changes

d. goal is to find and manage any life-threatening injuries

e. look, listen, and feel

f. creates a barrier between the Paramedic and potentially infectious materials

g. patient's eyes are open and he appears awake

h. assessment to assure the Paramedic's well-being

i. method of opening the airway for trauma patients

j. also referred to as "the look test" or "gut impression"

CHAPTER 14

THERAPEUTIC COMMUNICATIONS

Case Study

Your patient is an 11-year-old girl who has fallen from her skateboard and injured her left lower leg.

Decision Time

1. As you enter the scene, should you approach this patient differently than you would an adult patient with the same injury?

   _____

   _____

2. When you begin your initial assessment, you kneel at the patient's side within arm's reach. What is this amount of space considered in relation to the patient?

   _____

   _____

The patient's body language makes it clear that she is comfortable with where you have placed yourself, and she is communicating effectively.

3. What is the study of nonverbal behavior called?

   _____

   _____

In Retrospect . . .

4. What would have likely been the result if you had immediately moved to the patient's intimate space to examine her injury?

   _____

   _____

Practice Questions
Fill in the Blank

Complete each sentence by adding the appropriate word in the provided blanks.

1. Successful communication depends on the message being _____ and _____ correctly.

2. The overarching goal of _____ is to obtain clinically relevant information about the patient so that a diagnosis can be made and treatment offered.

3. A common obstacle to successful communication is the use of _____ terminology.

4. If applied correctly, therapeutic _____, such as hand holding, can help calm patients and transmit a message of compassion to the patient.

5. _____-ended questions allow a patient to give more thorough answers, whereas _____-ended questions result in fast responses and limited information.

6. When interviewing, avoid _____ questions, as they imply judgment.

7. The Paramedic should not give _____ assurances or advice.

8. Patients may exhibit self-protective behaviors, called _____ behaviors, which inhibit free dialogue with the Paramedic.

9. _____ and _____ are both excellent ways to ensure that the message sent was received correctly.

10. The Paramedic should strive for _____ _____, an ability to function effectively within the populations that he serves.

Matching

Match each term with its corresponding description.

_____ 11. personal space

_____ 12. kinesics

_____ 13. hermeneutics

_____ 14. cultural competence

_____ 15. culture

_____ 16. ethnocentrism

_____ 17. transmission

_____ 18. feedback

_____ 19. schizokinesis

_____ 20. proxemics

_____ 21. decode

_____ 22. self-awareness

_____ 23. open-ended question

_____ 24. body language

_____ 25. indirect statement

a. a view that one's own cultural practices and customs are superior

b. mechanism by which the Paramedic can assure that the message sent was properly received and decoded

c. explanation asked for by a Paramedic that is not constrained by a statement

d. ability to understand a message

e. transmission of a message by nonverbal visual cues

f. study of nonverbal behavior for communications

g. process of conveying a message

h. based on the concept of four spaces that surround a person

i. past painful experiences, unconsciously recalled by trigger words, that can elicit an autonomic nervous system response

j. the space in which most Paramedics interview patients for a history

k. culmination of life experiences in a locality or region that affects the way a person thinks and behaves

l. to allow patient to express self without restriction

m. having a conscious understanding of one's life influences and prejudices

n. an ability to function effectively within the populations that one serves

o. putting oneself in the patient's situation in order to understand the patient better

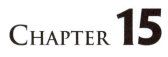

CHAPTER 15

HISTORY TAKING

Case Study

You are called to a suburban residence where a 54-year-old man is complaining of chest pain. After you verify that the scene is safe, you enter the patient's living room to find him clutching his chest in obvious distress.

Decision Time

1. Which of the mnemonics that you have learned is most appropriate to assess the patient's present illness?

   _____

   _____

2. Which of the mnemonics is most appropriate to assess a patient's past medical history?

   _____

   _____

Due to the patient's condition, you continue your assessment en route to the emergency room.

3. Which type of questions will provide the Paramedic with the most information?

   _____

   _____

After you arrive at the emergency room, you reflect on how you interviewed and assessed the patient.

In Retrospect . . .

4. How would you change your assessment if the patient was deaf and unable to hear your questions?

   _____

   _____

Practice Questions
Multiple Choice

Select the best answer for each of the following questions.

1. Which of the following greetings is an acceptable way of addressing a patient?
   a. Hi. I'm Mike, a Paramedic with the ambulance service. What's going on with you today?
   b. Hey, sweetie. I'm Mike, with the ambulance service. Are you feeling bad today?
   c. Hi. I'm Mike, a Paramedic with the ambulance service. What's wrong today, hon?
   d. Good morning, Mrs. Smith. I'm with the ambulance service. Are you sick today?

2. Your patient told you that he drank a couple of beers, then later tells you that he has consumed no alcoholic beverages. You remind him about his earlier statement and ask which is correct. This is an example of which interviewing technique?
   a. facilitation
   b. reflection
   c. clarification
   d. confrontation

3. You are assessing a patient who complains of chest pain when you ask, "You said it was a crushing pain." The patient replies, "It felt like my chest was in a vise." Which interviewing technique is represented here?
   a. facilitation
   b. reflection
   c. clarification
   d. confrontation

4. Which of the following is NOT a component of a comprehensive history?
   a. age
   b. insurance policy number
   c. chief concern
   d. psychosocial history

5. To what does the letter D in the mnemonic SAMPLED history refer?
   a. diagnosis
   b. diabetes
   c. depression
   d. advanced directives

Fill in the Blank

Complete each mnemonic by adding the appropriate word in the provided blanks.

OPQRST AS/PN

6. O = _____

7. P = _____

8. Q = _____

9. R = _____

10. S = _____

11. T = _____

12. AS = _____

13. PN = _____

AEIOU TIPS

14. A = _____

15. E = _____

16. I = _____

17. O = _____

18. U = _____

19. T = _____

20. I = _____

21. P = _____

22. S = _____

HAPI-SOCS

23. H = _____

24. A = _____

25. P = _____

26. I = _____

27. S = _____

28. O = _____

29. C = _____

30. S = _____

CHAPTER 16

PHYSICAL EXAMINATION AND SECONDARY ASSESSMENT

Case Study

You are called to assist an elderly nursing home patient who is nonambulatory. As you prepare to transport her, you realize that she has pressure ulcers on her buttocks.

Decision Time

1. What is another name for pressure ulcers?

   _____

   _____

2. Why are these especially dangerous?

   _____

   _____

3. What precautions should you take?

   _____

   _____

You don gloves and cover the patient's wounds with a sterile dressing.

4. What causes pressure ulcers?

   _____

   _____

5. How can pressure ulcers be prevented?

   _____

   _____

In Retrospect . . .

After this call, you think about the skin and all that it can tell you about someone's condition.

6. List at least three signs you can see on the skin, and what they mean.

_____

_____

Practice Questions

Multiple Choice

Select the best answer for each of the following questions.

1. Percussion of the chest reveals a hyperresonant sound. Which of the following is the most likely problem?
   a. pleural effusion
   b. pneumothorax
   c. myocardial infarction
   d. subcutaneous emphysema

2. What are vibrations palpated on the chest while the patient is speaking called?
   a. subcutaneous emphysema
   b. pleural effusion
   c. tactile fremitus
   d. none of the above

3. Which of the following is another term for bruising?
   a. tactile fremitus
   b. hernia
   c. jaundice
   d. ecchymosis

4. What term refers to the inner lining of the abdomen?
   a. ascites
   b. peritoneum
   c. visceral
   d. herniation

5. Which of the following is an easily treatable cause of altered mental status?
   a. hypoglycemia
   b. hyperglycemia
   c. transient ischemic attack
   d. hypoxemia

Matching

Terms

Match each term with its corresponding description.

_____ 6. pitting edema

_____ 7. systole

_____ 8. S3 and S4

_____ 9. S2

_____ 10. S1

_____ 11. vital signs

_____ 12. bradycardia

_____ 13. physical examination

_____ 14. capnography

_____ 15. palpation

_____ 16. systolic blood pressure

_____ 17. tripod position

_____ 18. capillary refill

_____ 19. inspection

_____ 20. pulse pressure

_____ 21. apical pulse

_____ 22. auscultation

_____ 23. pulse oximetry

_____ 24. cardiac output

_____ 25. aortic stenosis

a. end-tidal CO_2 detection

b. objectively measured characteristics of basic body function

c. non-invasive measurement of the percentage of hemoglobin in arterial blood that is bound to oxygen molecules

d. assessing the patient through listening

e. sign of severe respiratory distress

f. involves looking at the patient

g. adult heart rate under 60

h. assessing through touch

i. diastolic sounds that occur with ventricular filling

j. blood pressure measured during ventricular contraction

k. pulse rate at the chest

l. ventricular contraction

m. process by which a Paramedic performs an assessment of the patient from head to toe in an effort to detect signs associated with a disease or condition

n. corresponds to the closing of aortic and pulmonic valves

o. difference between systolic and diastolic pressures

p. volume of blood pumped out of the left ventricle in one minute

q. measure of the ability to perfuse the extremities with oxygenated blood

r. the amount of indentation produced when the edematous limb is pressed

s. condition in which leaflets of aortic valve become scarred and pathway through the valve narrows

t. corresponds to the closing of the mitral and tricuspid valve

Lung Sounds

Match each term with its corresponding description.

_____ 26. wheezing

_____ 27. rhonchi

_____ 28. consolidation

_____ 29. stridor

_____ 30. rales

a. crackles

b. coarse crackling in larger airways

c. high-pitched inspiratory sound heard with upper airway obstruction

d. high-pitched inspiratory sound found with asthma, COPD, and heart failure

e. bronchial sounds heard over periphery, unequal compared to same field on opposite lung

CHAPTER 17

CLINICAL DECISION MAKING AND TEAMWORK

Case Study

You have agreed to work an extra shift partly because you could use the extra money and partly because you will be working with veteran Paramedic Wanda Stubenaker. Stubenaker has a reputation for being sharp as a tack, tough as nails, and cool as a cucumber. You could learn a lot from Wanda.

Your first call is to attend to an 18-month-old who has dislocated her elbow—a classic nursemaid's elbow. Wanda expertly handles the scene, treats the girl and her family with tenderness, and reassures everyone on the scene with her quiet confidence. As you start to make up the cot for the next call, you ask Wanda about some of the decisions she made.

"I noticed that you didn't splint the dislocation," you say—almost in the form of a question. "Is that a problem?" she asks, with a hint of a smile on her face. "No. Well, maybe . . . ," you reply, not really knowing what to say.

Decision Time

1. Although the protocols call for the splinting of any swollen, deformed extremity, are there times when using a traditional splint may cause more damage than good?

   _____

   _____

Wanda smiles and tells you that it is okay to ask why she didn't splint the girl's arm. In her calm, easy manner, she explains that the best splint for the situation was the little girl being held in her mother's arms. "If I had tried to take the little girl from her mother, we could have caused more damage than good," she says. "Remember that the first rule of medicine is to do no harm. That's what we did by allowing Mom to hold the little girl."

2. Is this a case of good clinical decision making or simply reckless negligence?

   _____

   _____

Wanda compliments you for having the courage to ask the question, and tells you that as you gain experience and work with experienced Paramedics, you too will develop clinical judgment. "That doesn't mean taking shortcuts or ignoring what you learned in class," says Wanda. "What it does mean is that with experience, you can use that experience to better care for your patient. Remember that protocols assume that one patient's situation is the same or similar to another patient's condition in the same situation." She continues, "If that were a 30-year-old or perhaps even a 3-year-old, we could have splinted the dislocation without causing further damage. However, Mom had the elbow effectively splinted in her arms, the patient remained calm throughout transport, and we transported the patient without any further injury or distress."

In Retrospect . . .

3. What did you learn in just your first call with Wanda?

_____

_____

4. How would you like to have a Paramedic like Wanda that you could learn from at your service?

_____

_____

Practice Questions

Short Answer

Write a brief answer to each of the following questions.

1. Describe what makes the out-of-hospital environment different from any other.

_____

_____

2. Describe the limitations of the use of protocols, standing orders, and patient care algorithms.

_____

_____

3. What are the components of critical thinking?

_____

_____

4. How does a Paramedic develop medical intelligence?

_____

_____

5. What is a symptom complex?

_____

_____

Fill in the Blank

Complete each sentence by adding the appropriate word in the provided blanks.

6. The process of assessment and treatment planning is called _____ decision making.

7. The systematic approach to investigating a problem and coming to a decision based upon past experience and medical knowledge is called medical _____.

8. A collection of symptoms that characterize a condition or state is called a _____.

9. A _____ is a physiological deviation from a normal homeostasis.

10. The general assessment of the patient's condition is termed the _____ impression.

11. The Japanese term that means continuous performance improvement is _____.

12. _____ are a set of mandatory behaviors meant to be applied in specific clinical conditions.

13. The process of assessment, treatment, and reassessment is consistent with the quality improvement cycle: plan, do, _____, act.

14. To determine whether an emergency call is medical or trauma in nature, the Paramedic must consider the _____ of injury or the _____ of the illness.

15. The initial impression is used in conjunction with the primary assessment to determine if the patient is _____ or _____.

Matching

Match each term with its corresponding description.

_____ 16. garbage can diagnosis

_____ 17. mechanism of injury

_____ 18. Gestalt

_____ 19. defensive medicine

_____ 20. palliative

_____ 21. rules out

_____ 22. predictable injury pattern

_____ 23. Ockham's razor

_____ 24. nature of illness

_____ 25. paradigm blindness

a. the unwillingness to consider alternatives to patient care

b. a way of seeing a pattern in the observation of the patient as a whole

c. use of random tests to limit liability

d. supportive care

e. hasty field diagnosis that is broad and over-generalized

f. all things being equal, the simplest solution tends to be best

g. suggests trauma

h. characteristic injury

i. eliminates

j. suggests that the call is medical

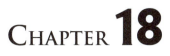

CHAPTER **18**

COMMUNICATIONS

Case Study

The call taker at the public safety access point (PSAP) answers the 9-1-1 call for help. "Help me, please," says the little girl. "My mommy is sleeping and I can't wake her up." The call taker dispatches the nearest law enforcement, fire, and EMS units, and continues the conversation with the little girl. The communications specialist learns that the little girl, Ellie, is 5 years old and came into the kitchen from her bedroom to find her mother collapsed on the floor. She has been unable to arouse her mother.

While you are en route, dispatch tells you what has happened and is happening on the scene. She tells you that Ellie can see her mother's chest rising and falling, and that her skin color is normal.

Decision Time

1. How will the information the dispatcher was able to gather before you arrived help you to prepare for the call?

_____

_____

Law enforcement and fire service personnel arrive before you and report that Ellie was incorrect—that her mother was not breathing. They start ventilating the patient and relay the message that the patient appears to have had a seizure. In addition, her tongue is bleeding.

2. How do the communications from first responders to the scene help you to prepare for the call?

_____

_____

In Retrospect . . .

3. Describe how the modern 9-1-1 and communications system helps you to provide better care.

_____

_____

Practice Questions
Short Answer

Write a brief answer to each of the following questions.

1. What is the primary advantage of using plain English over 10-codes?

_____

_____

2. What causes electrical interference in ECG tracings?

_____

_____

3. What was one of the earliest public safety uses of radio?

_____

_____

4. Why are satellite phones especially useful during disasters?

_____

_____

5. Where was the first 9-1-1 call made?

_____

_____

Fill in the Blank

Complete each sentence by adding the appropriate word in the provided blanks.

6. The _____ phase of communication in an EMS incident is a call received at a centralized communications center or public access point.

7. The second phase of emergency communications is the _____ and response phase.

8. The Communications Act of 1934 granted the Federal _____ Commission control over all civilian use of radios.

9. Approximately 96% of the United States is covered by the _____ system.

10. Technology allows Paramedics to use personal _____ assistants during calls to gather, transmit, and receive critical patient information.

Matching

Match each term with its corresponding description.

_____ 11. echo technique

_____ 12. duplex

_____ 13. alert report

_____ 14. squelch control

_____ 15. simplex

_____ 16. Federal Communications Commission

_____ 17. amplitude modulation (AM)

_____ 18. 9-1-1

_____ 19. cell phone

_____ 20. interference

_____ 21. multiplex

_____ 22. frequency modulation (FM)

_____ 23. AMPLE

_____ 24. repeater

_____ 25. scanner

a. universal emergency number used in the United States

b. reduces the amount of signal received between transmissions

c. has control over the civilian use of radios

d. extraneous electromagnetic energy heard on the radio

e. low-powered wireless transmitters that work within close proximity to a tower

f. radio waves modified by changing the speed of the wave

g. permits the transmission of audio signals and data

h. allows for communication in one direction at a time

i. radios that pick up, amplify, and then retransmit a radio transmission

j. uses two frequencies—one to transmit and one to receive—so that the operator can talk and listen at the same time

k. multiband receivers that monitor several radio frequencies

l. radio waves modified by changing the height of the wave

m. letting the receiving facility know you are en route

n. the act of repeating a medical order back verbatim

o. can be useful for organizing the patient's medical history

CHAPTER 19

DOCUMENTATION

Case Study

You are working your normal shift when the dispatcher asks you to return to quarters. When you arrive, you are met by a sheriff's deputy, who serves you with a subpoena to appear in court with patient care records for a motor vehicle collision that you worked more than two years ago. Although you have never been summoned to court before, you are most distressed by the fact that you do not even remember the call. You visit your supervisor's office to ask her advice. "Don't worry," she says. "It'll be okay. The good news is that you are not listed as a defendant—you are simply a witness."

Decision Time

1. Why is it not important that you remember the call?

Your supervisor helps to retrieve the PCR for you, and suggests that you review it carefully before your court date. Your supervisor explains, "You have been called to testify as a witness by either the plaintiff's or defendant's counsel," she says. "Whoever called you as a witness hopes that you will help their case. The other side may try to discredit you and your testimony," she said.

2. What is your best defense against being discredited?

One week before the court date you are notified that the case has been settled out of court, and you will not be needed to testify. You breathe a sigh of relief and reflect on the importance of an accurate patient care report.

In Retrospect . . .

3. Why is a complete and accurate patient care report so important to assure a clear legal document?

4. Other than the legal aspects of the patient care report, why is the PCR important?

Practice Questions

Multiple Choice

Select the best answer for each of the following questions.

1. Which of the following is an EMS-specific documentation method?
   a. SOAP notes
   b. OPQRST
   c. CHEATED
   d. progress notes

2. In the CHART method of EMS documentation, an additional I and E were added at the end. What does the I represent?
   a. interview
   b. intervention
   c. inventory
   d. in service

3. In the CHART method of EMS documentation, what does the letter R stand for?
   a. radiation of pain
   b. responders' names
   c. Rx prescription
   d. race

4. In the CHEATED method of EMS documentation, what does the letter D stand for?
   a. disposition
   b. diagnosis
   c. documentation
   d. none of the above

5. Which of the following is a chronological description of the development of the patient's present illness?
   a. symptom pattern
   b. history of present illness
   c. progress notes
   d. all of the above

Fill in the Blank

Complete each sentence by adding the appropriate word in the provided blanks.

6. Patient care documentation is a record of _____ findings and observations of the patient's health obtained through examination.

7. Since it may be used in the future by physicians and allied health professionals in a continuum of patient care, the patient care report is part of the _____ record.

8. Because it may be used in a court case, the PCR is a _____ record.

9. To assure clear copies, the Paramedic should use _____ ink on patient care reports.

10. Placing a single diagonal line across any open areas of the PCR is called a _____ -out.

Matching

Match each term with its corresponding description.

_____ 11. exposure report

_____ 12. LMP

_____ 13. sign out

_____ 14. SOAP notes

_____ 15. P in AMPLE

_____ 16. forced fields

_____ 17. NAD

_____ 18. NKDA

_____ 19. side rails up times two

_____ 20. constitutional symptoms

_____ 21. triage tag

_____ 22. master problem list

_____ 23. past medical history

_____ 24. M in AMPLE

_____ 25. detailed physical examination

a. no apparent distress

b. often the final line of documentation on the PCR

c. one of the earliest standardized documentation formats

d. past medical history

e. head-to-toe exam

f. general systemic reactions to illness

g. list of medical conditions for which a patient has been treated

h. medications

i. mandatory fields in an electronic document that cannot be skipped

j. filed separately from PCR

k. often documented by using AMPLE

l. no known drug allergies

m. placing time, date, and initials after the last entry

n. often only documentation completed by Paramedic in multi-casualty incident

o. last menstrual period

CHAPTER 20

AIRWAY ANATOMY AND PHYSIOLOGY

Case Study

You are called to care for a 3-month-old who is not breathing and is cyanotic. You open the patient's airway and look, listen, and feel for breathing. There is no breathing, so you apply positive pressure ventilation.

Decision Time

1. Why are pediatric patients more susceptible than adults to gastric distention?

   _____

   _____

2. How can you avoid causing gastric distention in a patient?

   _____

   _____

The patient has a pulse, and after just a few breaths of positive pressure ventilation his color improves.

3. What other anatomic airway differences exist between pediatric and adult patients?

   _____

   _____

In Retrospect . . .

Since the patient improved so quickly, you did not have to use any advanced airway techniques.

4. What is the most likely pathway to death for children?

   _____

   _____

Practice Questions
Fill in the Blank

Complete each sentence by adding the appropriate word in the provided blanks.

1. The openings of the _____ and _____ define the beginning of the airway.

2. Anatomically, the passage from the nare to the _____ is a straight line parallel to the roof of the mouth.

3. When the facial bones and the bones of the skull develop in the fetus, small air pockets called _____ form.

4. The _____ is able to humidify and filter inhaled air.

5. The lower jaw, or _____, articulates with the temporal bones at the temporomandibular joints.

6. The _____ and _____ are areas of common passage for food and respiratory gasses.

7. The _____ are the posterior-most structures of the laryngeal opening.

8. The _____ cartilage is the large, anterior, shield-like cartilage structure that forms the majority of the anterior portion of the larynx.

9. The open space below the laryngeal opening and superior to the vocal cords is called the _____.

10. The _____ _____ are composed of mucosal folds overlying ligaments, cartilages, and muscles.

Matching

Match each term with its corresponding description.

_____ 11. inspiratory capacity

_____ 12. vocal cords

_____ 13. surfactant

_____ 14. accessory muscles

_____ 15. diaphragm

_____ 16. carina

_____ 17. tidal volume

_____ 18. true ribs

_____ 19. valecula

_____ 20. intercostal muscles

_____ 21. right mainstem bronchus

_____ 22. thyroid gland

_____ 23. minute ventilation

_____ 24. intrinsic and extrinsic laryngeal muscles

_____ 25. acinus

a. fluid that decreases the surface tension of the alveoli and prevents them from collapsing during expiration

b. volume of gas that passes through the lungs in a minute

c. sac-like part of the lung supplied by a single terminal bronchiole

d. attach ribs to each other

e. largest muscle involved in inspiration

f. highly vascular, "H" shaped structure that lies along the sides of the larynx and upper trachea

g. used during active breathing

h. first seven ribs

i. volume of a normal breath

j. space formed between the anterior–superior surface of the epiglottis and the posterior base of the tongue

k. tidal volume plus the inspiratory reserve volume

l. more acutely angled bronchus

m. responsible for the gag reflex

n. area at which the lower airway splits into two mainstem bronchi

o. responsible for the production of speech and sound

CHAPTER 21

THE ALGORITHMIC APPROACH TO AIRWAY MANAGEMENT

Case Study #1

Your patient is a 54-year-old male who is found unresponsive. The scene is safe, and you have taken body substance isolation.

Decision Time

1. What is your first step?

_____

_____

Your patient is not breathing.

2. What is your next step?

_____

_____

When you attempt to ventilate the patient, the breaths will not go in.

3. What is your next action?

_____

_____

This time the breaths go in.

4. What would you have done if the breaths had not gone in?

_____

_____

In Retrospect . . .

5. How does the airway algorithm help you to care for your patient?

_____

_____

Case Study #2

It is a sunny Sunday afternoon in the late summer when you are called to a possible drowning at a private residence. You arrive on the scene and are summoned to the pool in the back yard. Your patient is a toddler who was found unconscious at poolside. His mother is holding him, limp and lifeless, in her arms. She is clearly distraught both at the condition of her 2-year-old and the fact that she let him get out of her sight long enough to apparently fall in the pool. "I was sitting on the edge of the pool with my feet in the water and he was sitting behind me playing with his cars and trucks. My cell phone rang, so I answered it. I noticed he wasn't moving and was turning blue," she said. As she blurts out this explanation, she thrusts him toward you in a desperate plea for your help.

Decision Time

1. Based on what the mother tells you, what should you suspect?

_____

_____

2. What actions will you take?

_____

_____

After performing back blows, a plastic piece of a truck is expelled, and the child begins to gasp for breath.

3. What should you do now?

_____

_____

The patient is now breathing and coughing. His airway appears clear and he is moving an adequate volume of air at an adequate rate. You further assess the patient and transport him to the emergency department for further evaluation.

In Retrospect . . .

4. Why is it automatically assumed that an unconscious, apneic child at poolside has drowned?

_____

_____

Why is it important that the Paramedic assess each patient so that something like an airway obstruction will not be missed?

Practice Questions
Multiple Choice

Select the best answer for each of the following questions.

1. Which of the following statements about algorithms is correct?
   a. The algorithm gives wide latitude in decision making.
   b. Algorithms provide an impetus for continuing action.
   c. Algorithms allow the Paramedic to determine what to do next.
   d. The algorithm requires the Paramedic to perform a specified set of actions in a particular order.

2. Which of the following statements about algorithms is NOT true?
   a. Without understanding standard algorithmic management and why it is important, the Paramedic may be unable to make a good decision to try an alternate approach.
   b. Algorithms are the tool of choice for dictating care in critically unstable prehospital patients.
   c. Classes such as Advanced Cardiac Life Support and Pediatric Advanced Life Support discourage the use of algorithms.
   d. The best algorithm can only serve as a guide; it is never a rigid set of rules that must be mechanically followed.

3. Which of the following airway algorithms may not fit well into the prehospital environment?
   a. Advanced Cardiac Life Support Airway Management
   b. Advanced Trauma Life Support Airway Management
   c. National Emergency Airway Management Course
   d. American Society of Anesthesiologists Difficult Airway Algorithm

4. Which of the following is NOT an indication for definitive airway control?
   a. failure to oxygenate
   b. failure to ventilate
   c. history of COPD
   d. nonpatent airway

5. You perform an initial assessment on your patient, and find that her airway is not patent. What is your first intervention?
   a. use of simple airway maneuvers
   b. application of oxygen
   c. jaw thrust
   d. attempt to ventilate

6. Your patient is cyanotic. Which of the following actions will you take FIRST?
   a. apply high-flow oxygen
   b. question patient about past medical history
   c. assess the patency of the airway
   d. intubate

7. Which of the following may be the least invasive method to treat a hypoxic patient?
   a. administration of Narcan
   b. positive pressure ventilation
   c. administration of D50
   d. administration of O_2

8. Which of the following statements about BLS and ALS skills is correct?
   a. Paramedics provide ALS interventions only.
   b. EMTs provide BLS interventions only.
   c. Paramedics must perform excellent non-intubating skills prior to performing intubating skills.
   d. Airway skills may be divided into BLS and ALS, with a clear division of duties between the EMT and Paramedic.

9. How quickly does hypoxic brain death occur after the patient becomes apneic?
   a. 4 to 6 minutes
   b. 6 to 10 minutes
   c. 10 to 15 minutes
   d. immediately

10. Which of the following conditions require emergency transportation?
    a. unmanageable airway
    b. uncontrollable bleeding
    c. complicated delivery
    d. all of the above

Short Answer

Write a brief answer for each of the following questions.

11. There will be times when a patient's airway cannot be established on the first attempt. What should be done in this circumstance?

   _____

   _____

12. What should you do if a second attempt to open the airway and ventilate the patient is unsuccessful?

_____

_____

13. The National Association of EMS Physicians advocates that the first intubation attempt is the best one, as each attempt may cause edema, bleeding, and patient deterioration. What can you do to assure that your first attempt is the best one?

_____

_____

14. According to the National Association of EMS Physicians, what four actions meet the definition of an intubation attempt?

_____

_____

15. How should intubation be confirmed?

_____

_____

16. Describe the role of algorithms in airway management.

_____

_____

17. What are the five situations that call for active airway or respiratory management?

_____

_____

18. What should you consider as a potential problem when presented with a patient who is unresponsive, but not in cardiac or respiratory arrest?

_____

_____

19. List several circumstances in which you would provide emergency transport.

_____

_____

20. Your patient is not breathing. You open the airway using the head-tilt, chin-lift method and attempt to ventilate using a bag-valve-mask. The air won't go in. What should you do?

_____

_____

21. How should you secure an endotracheal tube?

_____

_____

22. What are the advantages to using blind insertion airway devices?

_____

_____

23. What should you suspect if you are unable to ventilate a patient who is not intubated?

_____

_____

24. What should you suspect if you are unable to ventilate a patient who is intubated?

_____

_____

25. If your patient has an open airway, is protecting his own airway, and is adequately oxygenating and ventilating, what should you do?

_____

_____

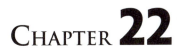

CHAPTER 22

NON-INTUBATING AIRWAY MANAGEMENT

Case Study

Your patient is a 54-year-old male who is found unresponsive. The scene is safe, and you have taken body substance isolation. You open the patient's airway with the head-tilt, chin-lift method and check for breathing. Your patient is not breathing, so you ventilate using a bag-valve-mask. When the breaths won't go in, you reposition the patient's head and try again. This time, the breaths go in. The patient has a pulse.

Decision Time

1. What airway adjunct can you use to help maintain the patient's airway?

   _____

   _____

Your patient does not have a gag reflex so you place an oropharyngeal airway.

2. While ventilating with a bag-valve-mask, how can you decrease the risk of gastric distention?

   _____

   _____

Although endotracheal intubation is the "gold standard" in airway management, intubation is of no use without excellent basic life support skills.

In Retrospect . . .

3. How can you assure that your basic airway skills are sharp?

   _____

   _____

Practice Questions
Fill in the Blank

Complete each sentence by adding the appropriate word in the provided blanks.

1. Quoting the 1994 EMT-Basic National Standard Curriculum, "a patient without an _____ is a dead patient."

2. The most important airway skills are the _____ skills.

3. Any patient in need of active airway management or ventilatory support is in need of supplemental _____.

4. Administering supplemental oxygen replaces _____ in the dead space of the lungs with oxygen.

5. Supplemental oxygen can _____ (increase or decrease) myocardial oxygen demand.

6. An oxygen D cylinder holds _____ liters of oxygen.

7. An oxygen E cylinder holds _____ liters of oxygen.

8. An M cylinder holds _____ liters of oxygen.

9. Large volumes of oxygen may be stored in a small space using concentrated _____ oxygen.

10. To deliver oxygen to the patient, you must first lower the pressure using a _____.

11. Oxygen delivery is measured in _____ per minute.

12. Transport ventilators typically operate at _____ PSI.

13. The simple face mask can deliver 40% to 60% FiO_2 at _____ liters per minute.

14. The demand valve regulator attached to a 50 PSI source will deliver _____% FiO_2.

15. The oral airway may stimulate a _____ _____.

Matching

Match each term with its corresponding description.

_____ 16. continuous positive airway pressure

_____ 17. preoxygenation

_____ 18. venturi mask

_____ 19. pulse oximetry

_____ 20. oropharyngeal airway

_____ 21. pocket mask

_____ 22. cricoid pressure

_____ 23. nasopharyngeal airway

_____ 24. tracheal intubation

_____ 25. head-tilt, chin-lift

a. allows Paramedic to monitor oxygenation during procedures

b. considered the gold standard of airway management

c. delivers a precise percentage of oxygen

d. may decrease gastric distention during positive pressure ventilation

e. displaces the soft palate anteriorly, improving airflow through the upper airway

f. capable of delivering 17% oxygen

g. may stimulate a gag reflex

h. increases the diffusion gradient of oxygen into the plasma and provides a reservoir of oxygen in the lungs

i. technique of choice for opening the airway in a non-trauma patient

j. assures that the airway pressure in all phases of the respiratory cycle is above zero

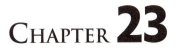

CHAPTER 23

INTUBATING AIRWAY MANAGEMENT

Case Study

Your patient is a 54-year-old male who is found unresponsive. The scene is safe, and you have taken body substance isolation. You open the airway with the head-tilt, chin-lift method and check for breathing. Your patient is not breathing, so you ventilate using a bag-valve-mask. When the breaths won't go in, you reposition the patient's head and try again. This time, the breaths go in. The patient has a pulse. You insert an oropharyngeal airway and continue to ventilate using a bag-valve-mask.

Decision Time

1. What adjunct can be used to help secure the patient's airway?

   _____

   _____

2. What are the advantages to using the endotracheal tube?

   _____

   _____

You prepare to intubate by gathering all of your equipment and preoxygenating your patient.

3. What equipment will you need for endotracheal intubation?

   _____

   _____

The intubation goes very smoothly, and you check tube placement by auscultation. You hear no gastric sounds but instead equal breath sounds.

4. What other method must you use to ensure correct placement?

   _____

   _____

In Retrospect . . .

5. Why is it so important to prepare in advance for the intubation?

   _____

   _____

Practice Questions

Fill in the Blank

Complete each sentence by adding the appropriate word in the provided blanks.

1. The distal end of the endotracheal tube features a _____ eye, which decreases the opportunity for tube obstruction.

2. The Esophageal Tracheal Combitube (ETC) is a _____ lumen device that is placed in the esophagus.

3. The Esophageal Tracheal Combitube (ETC) is demonstrated to cause _____ (less or more) C-spine movement than conventional endotracheal intubation.

4. Lighted stylettes are _____ stylettes with a bright light source.

5. The tip of the Macintosh blade is designed to fit into the _____.

Matching

Match each term with its corresponding description.

_____ 6. digital intubation

_____ 7. complication of endotracheal intubation

_____ 8. nasogastric tube

_____ 9. tracheobronchial suctioning

_____ 10. disadvantage of endotracheal intubation

_____ 11. Miller blade

_____ 12. LEMON law

_____ 13. laryngoscope

_____ 14. elastic gum bougie

_____ 15. Esophageal Tracheal Combitube

_____ 16. BURP technique

_____ 17. nasotracheal intubation

_____ 18. colorimetric device

_____ 19. pediatric endotracheal tube

_____ 20. endotracheal tube

_____ 21. MacIntosh blade

_____ 22. stylet

_____ 23. DOPE

_____ 24. laryngeal mask airway

_____ 25. advantage of endotracheal intubation

a. dual lumen airway device

b. straight laryngoscope blade

c. helps to remember causes of problem intubations

d. primary device used to visualize the larnyx

e. air is not filtered, warmed, or humidified by upper airway

f. curved laryngoscope blade

g. does not cause gastric distention

h. blind airway device designed for use in the operating room

i. most common CO_2 detector

j. provides rigidity to the endotracheal tube

k. method of improving laryngoscopic view

l. method of evaluating patient for potentially difficult intubation

m. placing an endotracheal tube through the nostril of the patient into the trachea

n. direct suctioning of the tracheobronchial tree

o. provides a conduit for oxygenation and ventilation between the patient's lungs and the ventilator

p. used to evacuate air from the stomach

q. directed through the vocal cords and into the trachea to serve as a guide for the endotracheal tube

r. typically uncuffed

s. includes laryngeal swelling and vocal cord damage

t. blind intubation accomplished with tactile placement

CHAPTER 24

MEDICATION-FACILITATED INTUBATION

Case Study

Your patient is a 24-year-old male who has crashed his motorcycle into a bridge abutment on a rural highway. The nearest hospital is 30 minutes away and the nearest trauma center is two hours away by ground. Your patient was not wearing a helmet, and has sustained a good deal of facial trauma. He is combative, does not respond to your commands, and is having severe difficulty breathing, with respiratory rate of 44, shallow and labored.

Decision Time

1. Is this patient a candidate for rapid sequence intubation (RSI)?

   _____

   _____

2. Is this patient a candidate for helicopter transport?

   _____

   _____

You see that you cannot effectively control the patient's airway with him in his current condition, so you decide to utilize RSI.

3. What are the nine P's of RSI?

   _____

   _____

You go through the nine P's of RSI, and successfully intubate the patient.

4. What are the components of post-intubation care?

   _____

   _____

In Retrospect . . .

5. How does the axiom, "the first (intubation) attempt is the best attempt" pertain to RSI?

   _____

   _____

Practice Questions

Short Answer

Write a brief answer to each of the following questions.

1. What two agents are commonly used as adjuncts to emergency rapid sequence intubation?

   _____

   _____

2. Why must extraordinary judgment be exercised before deciding to sedate and chemically paralyze a patient?

   _____

   _____

3. What two tools can be used to perform an airway evaluation before and during airway management?

   _____

   _____

4. Why should you preoxygenate the patient prior to intubation?

   _____

   _____

5. What post-intubation tasks should be performed after the tube is secured?

   _____

   _____

Matching

Rapid Sequence Intubation (RSI)

Place each of the nine P's of rapid sequence intubation (RSI) in the correct order.

_____ 6.	a.	pretreat
_____ 7.	b.	pass the tube
_____ 8.	c.	paralyze
_____ 9.	d.	preparation
_____ 10.	e.	post-intubation care
_____ 11.	f.	preoxygenate
_____ 12.	g.	pressure on the cricoid
_____ 13.	h.	predict the degree of difficulty
_____ 14.	i.	position (confirm) and secure

Pharmacological Intubation Adjuncts

Match each term with its corresponding description.

_____ 15. malignant hyperthermia

_____ 16. succinylcholine

_____ 17. sedative agents

_____ 18. ketamine

_____ 19. midazolam

_____ 20. fentanyl

_____ 21. etomidate

_____ 22. narcotics

_____ 23. benzodiazepines

_____ 24. neuromuscular blockers

_____ 25. vecuronium

a. highly potent synthetic opioid

b. hypnotic and amnestic

c. most commonly used NMBA in prehospital environment

d. most commonly used medications for sedation in emergency airway management

e. block transmission of nerve impulses to skeletal muscle

f. has minimal respiratory depression even at high doses

g. absolute contraindication to the use of succinylcholine

h. short-acting benzodiazepine that can be used as a sole agent to facilitate intubation

i. medications that decrease a patient's level of consciousness and an amnesia to events

j. most commonly used depolarizing neuromuscular blocker

k. able to induce a profound state of sedation

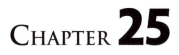

CHAPTER **25**

VENTILATION

Case Study

You are called to a manufacturing facility where a young female has "passed out." You are met at the door by her supervisor who rolls his eyes and tells you that she is just doing this to get out of work. "She has done it before," he says. "Probably trouble at home and she just doesn't want to be here. Just use some of those smelling salts so I can get everyone back to work," he continues.

Your patient is supine on the floor near the break room, attended to by some of her friends. She responds with a moan to painful stimulus.

Decision Time

1. Does the patient's history of "passing out" on the job before impact how you will assess her?

   _____

   _____

2. Why is it important to keep an open mind and assess the patient based on her current condition?

   _____

   _____

The patient's friend tells you that prior to passing out, the patient clutched her chest, said she couldn't breathe, and had very fast and shallow respirations. Although you are starting to believe that your patient hyperventilated and passed out, it is imperative that you consider all signs and symptoms.

3. What are some of the possible causes of hyperventilation?

   _____

   _____

In Retrospect . . .

Although hyperventilation can be caused as a response to fear, anxiety, or emotional stressors, it can also be caused by a number of physiological causes.

4. How does knowledge of acid–base balance help you to understand at a cellular level what might be happening with your patient?

   _____

   _____

5. Since you probably do not have the benefit of arterial blood gas analysis in the prehospital setting, why is it important that you understand acid–base balance?

   _____

   _____

Practice Questions

Multiple Choice

Select the best answer for each of the following questions.

1. Which of the following is a definition of respiration?
   a. movement of respiratory gasses in and out of the lungs
   b. the chemical processes by which an organism supplies its cells and tissues with the oxygen needed for metabolism and relieves them of the carbon dioxide formed in energy-producing reactions
   c. neither a nor b
   d. both a and b

2. Which of the following is NOT a component of respiration?
   a. absorption of oxygen into the cells
   b. utilization of oxygen to make energy
   c. inhalation of carbon dioxide
   d. movement of oxygen into the bloodstream

3. What percent of room air does oxygen comprise?
   a. 15%
   b. 16%
   c. 21%
   d. 24%

4. What percentage of oxygen that enters the bloodstream is dissolved into the plasma?
   a. 3%
   b. 5%
   c. 8% to 10%
   d. 16%

5. What is the typical oxygen saturation of venous blood?
   a. 55%
   b. 75%
   c. 86%
   d. 97%

6. What is the typical oxygen saturation of arterial blood?
   a. 55%
   b. 75%
   c. 86%
   d. 97%

7. Which of the following is a factor that increases the ability to bind oxygen to hemoglobin?
   a. increased CO_2
   b. increased 2,3-BPG
   c. increased pH
   d. increased temperature

8. Carbon dioxide reacts with water to form which of the following?
   a. carbonic anhydrase
   b. carbolic acid
   c. carbonic acid
   d. carbolic anhydrase

9. What is the normal pH range of human blood?
   a. 7.00 to 8.00
   b. 7.25 to 7.35
   c. 7.35 to 7.45
   d. 7.45 to 8.45

10. Which of the following body systems is NOT a key player in acid–base balance?
    a. renal system
    b. respiratory system
    c. gastrointestinal system
    d. buffer system

Fill in the Blank

Complete each sentence by adding the appropriate word in the provided blanks.

11. Each red blood cell contains approximately 270 million _____ molecules.

12. When a hemoglobin molecule attaches to at least one oxygen molecule, it is called _____.

13. Carbon dioxide is _____ times more soluble than oxygen in the blood for the same partial pressure.

14. A molecule that has a proton which is not orbited by a paired negatively charged atomic particle attached to it is also called an _____.

15. The pH scale ranges from _____ to 14.

16. A neutral pH is _____.

17. Excessive acid in the system is called _____.

18. The blood becomes _____ if the pH rises above 7.45.

19. Pulse _____ is a non-invasive measure of the percentage of hemoglobin sites in the red blood cells that are bound to oxyhemoglobin.

20. A normal SpO_2 is between _____% and 100%.

Matching

Match each term with its corresponding description.

_____ 21. normal blood pH

_____ 22. acid load

_____ 23. erythrocyte

_____ 24. pyrexia

_____ 25. pH scale

_____ 26. bicarbonate

_____ 27. acidosis

_____ 28. buffer

_____ 29. respiratory alkalosis

_____ 30. alkalosis

a. fever

b. excessive amounts of acid in the tissues

c. blood pH of less than 7.35

d. rendered neutral

e. red blood cell

f. 7.35 to 7.45

g. occurs when ventilation is greater than the body's CO_2 production

h. ranges from 0 to 14

i. blood pH of greater than 7.45

j. most common chemical buffer in the body

CHAPTER **26**

PRINCIPLES OF MEDICATION ADMINISTRATION

Case Study

You are called to care for a patient who complains of chest pain. Your patient is a 58-year-old male who smokes two packs of cigarettes per day. He has a history of cardiovascular disease and chronic bronchitis. As you load the patient into the ambulance, you determine that pharmacological therapy is indicated.

Decision Time

1. What question should you ask any patient before you administer any type of medication?

   _____

   _____

2. What route of administration will provide the fastest effect?

   _____

   _____

During your assessment, you find that the patient has a nitroglycerin patch.

3. What is the route of administration for this medication?

   _____

   _____

In Retrospect . . .

4. Does the presence of the nitroglycerin patch impact the amount of nitroglycerin that you administer?

   _____

   _____

Practice Questions
Fill in the Blank

Complete each sentence by adding the appropriate word in the provided blanks.

1. Bioassay measurements are standardized through the use of _____ units.

2. The _____ route bypasses the gastrointestinal system.

3. Administration of medications through the gastrointestinal system is referred to as the _____ route.

4. The _____ route involves placing the medication between the patient's cheek and gum.

5. A large diameter tube sometimes used to evacuate the stomach after a suicide attempt is called an _____ tube.

6. It is the Paramedic's responsibility to choose the _____ drug and the _____ dose for the patient, and to administer it by the _____ route at the _____ time in order to achieve the optimal therapeutic effect.

7. The _____ system of measurement, which uses units of grain, is rarely used today.

8. Conversions of _____ measurements are based on a factor of 10.

9. The drug _____ is described as the amount of drug in 1 milliliter of a solution.

10. Drugs that are absorbed from the _____ avoid interaction by stomach acids and intestinal enzymes.

Matching

Match each term with its corresponding description.

_____ 11. dry powder inhalers

_____ 12. transdermal

_____ 13. optic medications

_____ 14. otic medications

_____ 15. capsule

_____ 16. lozenges

_____ 17. suspension

_____ 18. spirits

_____ 19. magmas

_____ 20. syrups

_____ 21. emulsions

_____ 22. lotions

_____ 23. tinctures

_____ 24. tablet

_____ 25. sublingual

a. placed under the tongue

b. medicines intended to dissolve in the mouth

c. medicines mixed with sugar and water

d. powdered drugs with particles so large that they are visible when mixed in water

e. medicinal substances which are dissolved in alcohol

f. solid drug pulverized into microfine particles for inhalation

g. medicinal powder placed within a gelatin casing

h. medicines that remain as finely pulverized particles floating in the liquid

i. finely pulverized particles placed in oils

j. liquids that have a volatile oil that evaporates at room temperature and leaves a distinct odor in the air

k. designed for absorption into the skin

l. dry medicinal powder compressed into a pill shape

m. medications meant for the skin and placed in water

n. medications applied into the ear

o. medications topically applied to the eyes

Chapter 27

INTRAVENOUS ACCESS

Case Study

You arrive at a downtown office where bystanders are performing CPR on a 57-year-old man. You assess the patient and find that he is indeed pulseless and apneic.

Decision Time

1. Is IO a viable option for this patient?

   _____

   _____

2. Which common cardiac arrest medications can you give via the IO line?

   _____

   _____

You establish an IO line and administer epinephrine and amiodarone via IO infusion.

3. What is a disadvantage to the use of IO?

   _____

   _____

In Retrospect . . .

4. What are some of the risks of IO infusion?

   _____

   _____

Practice Questions

Multiple Choice

Select the best answer for each of the following questions.

1. How much water does the adult human body contain?
   a. 10 liters
   b. 20 liters
   c. 30 liters
   d. 40 liters

2. Which of the following is NOT considered a body compartment?
   a. intravascular
   b. intracellular
   c. extracellular
   d. intercellular

3. Which of the following represents a concentrated quantity of medication injected within the intravascular space?
   a. trauma line
   b. bolus
   c. wide open
   d. intravenous line

4. Which of the following is NOT a reason for starting an IV?
   a. fluid replacement
   b. lifeline
   c. injecting medicine into central circulation
   d. fluid bolus

5. Which of the following is NOT a sign of hypovolemia?
   a. lackluster eyes
   b. thirst
   c. dry and cracked lips
   d. dry and furrowed tongue

6. What is the best replacement for lost blood?
   a. blood
   b. blood substitute
   c. crystalloids
   d. colloids

7. What percentage of salt does normal saline contain?
   a. 9%
   b. 0.99%
   c. 0.09%
   d. the same amount as blood

8. Which of the following fluids is NOT isotonic?
   a. D_5W
   b. normal saline
   c. half normal saline
   d. lactated Ringer's

9. What is the part of the IV administration set that pierces the fluid container?
   a. proximal connector
   b. distal end
   c. spike
   d. drip chamber

10. How many drops does it take to deliver 1 mL using a micro-drop set?
    a. 10
    b. 12
    c. 15
    d. 60

11. Which of the following will deliver the most fluid quickly?
    a. 14 gauge catheter using a micro-drop set
    b. 16 gauge catheter using a micro-drop set
    c. 18 gauge catheter using a macro-drop set
    d. 20 gauge catheter using a macro-drop set

12. Which of the following will deliver the most fluid quickly?
    a. 14 gauge catheter with a short micro-drop set
    b. 14 gauge catheter with a long micro-drop set
    c. 14 gauge catheter with a short macro-drop set
    d. 14 gauge catheter with a long macro-drop set

13. Which of the following is NOT an advantage of peripheral venous access?
    a. accessible during cardiovascular collapse
    b. compressible
    c. readily available
    d. relatively easy to perform

14. Which of the following IV catheters would be less likely to cause thrombophlebitis?
    a. 14 gauge
    b. 16 gauge
    c. 18 gauge
    d. 20 gauge

15. Which vein runs down the lateral aspect of the forearm and terminates proximal to the thumb?
    a. cephalic
    b. basilic
    c. femoral
    d. jugular

16. Which of the following is NOT a peripheral vein?
    a. cephalic
    b. basilic
    c. external jugular
    d. dorsal venous plexus

17. Which of the following patients would likely be the easiest to initiate on IV?
    a. 78-year-old female with CHF
    b. 45-year-old male who has undergone chemotherapy
    c. 45-year-old female with chest pain
    d. 78-year-old obese female

18. What condition exists when the body is unable to drain excess interstitial fluid out of the tissues, resulting in swelling of the affected limb?
    a. pitting edema
    b. lymphedema
    c. peripheral edema
    d. physiologic edema

19. What is one situation in which the Paramedic would specifically use a povidone-iodine solution instead of alcohol to prep an IV site?
    a. patient is allergic to alcohol
    b. drawing a blood alcohol sample
    c. patient is allergic to latex
    d. marking the location of the injection site

20. Which of the following is an indication for adult intraosseous placement?
    a. unable to start peripheral IV on first attempt
    b. cardiac arrest
    c. bilateral femur fractures
    d. helicopter transport

Short Answer

Write a brief answer to each of the following questions.

21. What is the single largest drawback to IO infusion?

   _____

   _____

22. Where can the IO needle be placed in the adult patient?

   _____

   _____

23. Why do infants and children sometimes have more difficulty tolerating a fluid overload than adults?

   _____

   _____

24. List at least four pre-existing medical conditions that can contribute to increased fluid loss.

   _____

   _____

25. What is the difference between crystalloids and colloids?

   _____

   _____

26. Describe what happens when a hypotonic solution is infused.

   _____

   _____

27. Regarding the intravenous drip set, what factors impact the speed and volume at which fluid is infused?

   _____

   _____

28. What is the advantage of using a larger bore IV catheter?

   _____

   _____

29. What is the advantage of using a smaller bore IV catheter?

   _____

   _____

30. What are some of the complications of IO access?

   _____

   _____

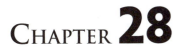

BLOOD PRODUCTS AND TRANSFUSION

Case Study

You are called to a local hospital to transport a trauma patient to a major medical center. The patient is receiving blood, which you will continue to monitor during the 30-minute trip.

Decision Time

1. What do you need to verify before transport?

   _____

   _____

2. As you assess your patient before transport, what should you check?

   _____

   _____

During the transfer, you monitor the flow of blood through the blood transfusion set.

3. What should you do if the unit of blood empties during transport?

   _____

   _____

The transport goes without difficulty. Upon arrival at the hospital, you complete your documentation and give a report to the receiving RN.

In Retrospect . . .

4. Why is it important to check the patient's temperature while blood is being transfused?

   _____

   _____

Practice Questions

Multiple Choice

Select the best answer for each of the following questions.

1. Which of the following is NOT one of the infectious diseases for which donated blood is tested?
   a. hepatitis A virus
   b. hepatitis B virus
   c. hepatitis C virus
   d. treponema pallidum

2. Which of the following is NOT one of the main solid components of blood?
   a. erythrocytes
   b. leukocytes
   c. hemocytoblast
   d. thrombocytes

3. Where are most of the coagulation factors located?
   a. pancreas
   b. liver
   c. spleen
   d. medulla oblongata

4. Which of the following are formed by removing the red blood cells and platelets from whole blood?
   a. packed red blood cells
   b. fresh frozen plasma
   c. cryoprecipitate
   d. platelets

5. Which of the following are formed by removing nearly all of the plasma from a unit of blood and adding a small volume of preservative to the unit?
   a. packed red blood cells
   b. fresh frozen plasma
   c. cryoprecipitate
   d. platelets

6. Which of the following is the protein portion of plasma made up of concentrated clotting factors?
   a. packed red blood cells
   b. fresh frozen plasma
   c. cryoprecipitate
   d. platelets

7. Which of the following terms refers to the clumping together of red blood cells?
   a. hemolysis
   b. transfusion
   c. agglutination
   d. none of the above

8. Your patient has type O blood. Which blood type(s) can he receive?
   a. A
   b. B
   c. AB
   d. O

9. Your patient has type B blood. Which blood type(s) can he receive?
   a. B and O
   b. A and O
   c. O
   d. B, AB, and O

10. Which blood type is considered the universal donor?
    a. A
    b. B
    c. AB
    d. O

Short Answer

Write a brief answer to each of the following questions.

11. What causes allergic reactions during blood transfusions?

_____

_____

12. How does transfusion associated circulatory overload occur?

_____

_____

13. Describe what causes an acute hemolytic reaction?

_____

_____

14. What is the major function of the red blood cells?

_____

_____

15. What is the major function of the white blood cells?

_____

_____

Fill in the Blank

Complete each sentence by adding the appropriate word in the provided blanks.

16. Platelets are part of the blood _____ process.

17. A unit of packed red blood cells will increase hemoglobin levels by _____ gm/dL.

18. Type AB blood is called the universal _____.

19. The patient should have vital signs recorded every _____ minutes during transfusion.

20. There are _____ major blood types.

Matching

Match each complete blood count (CBC) component to its normal range.

_____ 21. red blood cells

_____ 22. platelets

_____ 23. white blood cells

_____ 24. hematocrit

_____ 25. hemoglobin

a. 100,000 to 450,000 per mL

b. 13 to 16 g/dL (male); 12 to 15 g/dL (female)

c. 4.5 to 5.5 million per mL

d. 41% to 50% for males; 36% to 44% for females

e. 4,000 to 10,000 per mL

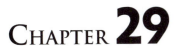
INTRODUCTION TO PHARMACOLOGY

Case Study

You respond to a residence to find an 82-year-old female patient who states that she has experienced dizziness for a little over a week. While conducting your assessment, you ask the patient about her medications. She tells you that her medications are in a bag on the kitchen counter. When you go into the kitchen to retrieve the bag, you find a large paper bag filled with at least 20 bottles, tubes, and boxes of medications.

Decision Time

1. Is it uncommon for elderly patients to take multiple medications?

_____

_____

2. Is there a good chance of medication errors when the patient takes that many medications?

_____

_____

En route to the hospital, the patient admits that she is unclear about what medications she is supposed to take, and that it is possible that she may have taken too much of some of her medications.

3. How could taking too much (or too little) of a medication cause untoward effects?

_____

_____

In Retrospect . . .

4. How could this situation be avoided in the future?

_____

_____

Practice Questions
Fill in the Blank

Complete each sentence by adding the appropriate word in the provided blanks.

1. When the decline of drug in the bloodstream reaches _____% of the original concentration, this is equivalent to the drug's half-life.

2. When the drug levels attain the targeted value, it has reached the _____ level.

3. Blood volume can have a dramatic impact on drug _____.

4. Drugs bind to certain substances in the body and, in doing so, form drug _____.

5. The difference between the amount administered and the amount that is bound and unavailable for use is called _____.

6. The drug's mechanism of _____ helps the Paramedic to understand how the cell will respond, how the organ is affected, and the total systemic response.

7. The _____ is the portion of a cell that attracts a certain molecule.

8. A cell receptor stimulator is also called a/an _____.

9. The drug's _____ is a measure of how the drug will realize its full intended effect.

10. _____ prevent enzymes from stimulating the metabolism of the cell.

Matching

Match each term with its corresponding description.

_____ 11. therapeutic index

_____ 12. Physician's Desk Reference

_____ 13. pharmacokinetics

_____ 14. first pass metabolism

_____ 15. drug

_____ 16. over-the-counter

_____ 17. therapeutic effect

_____ 18. generic name

_____ 19. side effects

_____ 20. chemical name

_____ 21. trade name

_____ 22. United States Pharmacopeia

_____ 23. prescription drugs

_____ 24. absorption

_____ 25. National Formulary

a. compendium of manufacturer's drug prescribing information which is usually found in a package insert

b. drug name listed in the USP

c. intended biological effect

d. name used to distinguish a patented drug

e. the ratio of the difference between the median effective dose and the median lethal dose

f. any material that is injected, ingested, inhaled, or absorbed into the body and is used for the diagnosis, treatment, or cure of a disease or condition

g. drug reference created by an independent non-governmental science-based public health organization

h. drugs that can contain an amount, or dose, of drug that can have serious side effects and require careful patient monitoring by a healthcare provider

i. the liver's actions upon the drugs

j. drugs sold to patients to self-treat minor illness

k. description of a drug according to its chemical makeup and molecular structure

l. manual that lists prescription medications

m. study of how drug absorption, distribution, detoxification, and elimination affect a drug's therapeutic value

n. first phase of a drug's life

o. unintended effects

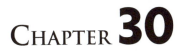

CHAPTER 30

PHARMACOLOGICAL INTERVENTIONS FOR CARDIOPULMONARY EMERGENCIES

Case Study

You respond to a call and find a 69-year-old male complaining of a "fluttering" in his chest. He denies a history of cardiovascular disease, and states that he feels like his heart is "about to leap from his chest." The patient's pulse rate is 200 and regular. His skin is pale, cool, and clammy. As you apply supplemental oxygen, your partner applies the cardiac monitor.

Decision Time

1. At first impression, is the patient stable or unstable?

   _____

   _____

2. What do you expect his blood pressure to be like?

   _____

   _____

You glance at the monitor, which reveals a wide-complex tachycardia—ventricular tachycardia—so you decide to get en route as you prepare an IV line.

3. According to the Vaughn–Williams classification, which classes of antidysrhythmic drugs may be effective on ventricular dysrhythmias?

   _____

   _____

In Retrospect . . .

4. Which medications carried in your EMS system might be effective for this patient? What other treatments might be indicated?

   _____

   _____

Practice Questions

Fill in the Blank

Complete each sentence by adding the appropriate word in the provided blanks.

1. Sympathomimetics, which are often either prodrugs or analogs of norepinephrine, share a common base molecule, and are called _____.

2. An alteration in the heart's rhythm is called a _____.

3. Parasympathetic nerves control narrowing the airway's lumen, called _____.

4. Class III drugs block _____ movement from the cell, lengthening the period of time in which the cell cannot respond to another stimulus.

5. _____ is a fibrous soluble protein that is found floating in the blood.

Matching

Terms

Match each term with its corresponding description.

_____ 6. acetylcholine

_____ 7. parasympathomimetic

_____ 8. sympathetic nervous system

_____ 9. fasciculations

_____ 10. anticholinergics

_____ 11. central nervous system

_____ 12. vagus nerve

_____ 13. antagonist

_____ 14. serotonin

_____ 15. peripheral nervous system

_____ 16. agonist

_____ 17. parasympathetic nervous system

_____ 18. nicotinic receptors

_____ 19. norepinephrine

_____ 20. resting membrane potential

a. chief neurotransmitter of the parasympathetic nervous system

b. neurotransmitter found primarily in intestinal tract, also found in platelets and brain

c. major parasympathetic nerve

d. increases gastric motility and stimulates erections in men

e. difference in electrical potential between outside and inside of the cell

f. consists of 12 cranial nerves and 31 spinal nerves

g. blocks the cell's ability to be stimulated

h. provides fight-or-flight response

i. blocks acetylcholine from binding to either muscarinic or nicotinic receptors

j. increases the neurotransmitter's ability to stimulate the cell's receptors

k. consists of the brain and spinal cord

l. chief neurotransmitter of the sympathetic system

m. transient fine muscle contractions seen after administration of a depolarizing neuromuscular blocker

n. cholinergic receptor located in the adrenal medulla

o. neurotransmitter that mimics the action of acetylcholine

Drug Types

Match each term with its corresponding description.

_____ 21. mucolytics

_____ 22. nitrates

_____ 23. vasopressors

_____ 24. diuretics

_____ 25. antihypertensives

_____ 26. antihyperlipidemics

_____ 27. antiplatelets

_____ 28. antidysrhythmics

_____ 29. fibrinolytics

_____ 30. corticosteroids

a. disassemble the fibrin clot

b. dilate the venous system, reducing blood return to the heart

c. thin the respiratory secretions

d. elevate blood pressure

e. control elevated lipid levels in the blood

f. alter platelet membranes, preventing aggregation, adherence, and vasoconstriction

g. decrease blood pressure

h. control cardiac disturbances

i. reduce swelling

j. cause increased loss of fluids and salts

CHAPTER 31

PHARMACOLOGICAL THERAPEUTICS FOR MEDICAL EMERGENCIES

Case Study

You are called to a local housing project where you find an unresponsive 34-year-old female. She is maintaining her own airway, breathing 20 times a minute, and has a pulse rate of 90. According to the patient's mother, she is diabetic and takes insulin daily. She said that her daughter came home earlier, seemed grouchy, and went to her bedroom. When called for dinner, she didn't answer, and you were called.

Decision Time

1. What condition do you expect the patient has?

   _____

   _____

2. What questions will you ask the patient's mother to try to determine if this is the patient's problem?

   _____

   _____

Your partner applies O$_2$ as you do a quick glucose test, which reads 40.

3. What pharmacological intervention is appropriate?

   _____

   _____

As you depart for the hospital, you start an IV and make sure that it is patent before you push the D50. Soon after you push the D50 and flush the line, the patient begins to arouse.

In Retrospect . . .

4. What might have disturbed your patient's glucose level?

   _____

   _____

Practice Questions

Multiple Choice

Select the best answer for each of the following questions.

1. Which of the following is NOT a component of the brainstem?
   a. cerebellum
   b. midbrain
   c. pons
   d. medulla oblongata

2. Which of the following parts of the brain is responsible for balance and muscular coordination?
   a. medulla
   b. cerebrum
   c. cerebellum
   d. pons

3. Which of the following is contained inside the cerebrum?
   a. white matter
   b. gray matter
   c. cerebral cortex
   d. pons

4. Capillaries have small gaps, called _____, that permit hormones, enzymes, and drugs to move into the interstitial space.
   a. astrocytes
   b. blastocytes
   c. slit junctions
   d. alveolar walls

5. Which of the following side effects do you NOT expect with sedatives?
   a. relaxation
   b. increased irritability
   c. decreased excitability
   d. reduced anxiety

6. Which of the following terms refer to an agent that reduces apprehension, fear, and anxiety?
   a. CNS depressant
   b. anxiolytic
   c. sedative
   d. paralytic

7. Which of the following is an example of an ultra-short acting barbiturate?
   a. phenobarbital
   b. secobarbital
   c. thiopental
   d. pentobarbital

8. How long is the intended pharmaceutical effect of long-acting barbiturates?
   a. 4 hours
   b. 8 hours
   c. 12 hours
   d. 24 hours

9. Which of the following is NOT an advantage of benzodiazepines over barbiturates?
   a. lethal dose is much higher for benzodiazepines than for barbiturates
   b. benzodiazepines have fewer side effects than barbiturates
   c. benzodiazepines have lower potential for abuse than barbiturates
   d. all benzodiazepines are short-acting, whereas some barbiturates are long-acting

106 Foundations of Paramedic Care Study Guide

© 2010 Cengage Learning. All Rights Reserved. May not be scanned, copied or duplicated, or posted to a publicly accessible website, in whole or in part.

10. Which of the following is an antidote for benzodiazepine?
    a. naloxone
    b. methadone
    c. flumazenil
    d. benzanil

Short Answer

Write a brief answer to each of the following questions.

11. Where in the body is insulin produced?

    _____

    _____

12. Why is an allergic reaction to injected insulin rare today?

    _____

    _____

13. What is the leading cause of blindness?

    _____

    _____

14. Describe type 1 diabetes.

    _____

    _____

15. How does syrup of ipecac work?

    _____

    _____

Matching

Match each term with its corresponding description.

_____ 16. ataxia

_____ 17. dyskinesia

_____ 18. patient-controlled analgesia

_____ 19. pain threshold

_____ 20. nociceptors

_____ 21. visceral pain

_____ 22. balanced anesthesia

_____ 23. neuromodulators

_____ 24. salicylate

_____ 25. analgesia

_____ 26. hydantoins

_____ 27. pre-induction agents

_____ 28. anesthesia

_____ 29. referred pain

_____ 30. nystagmus

a. acute pain from the internal organs

b. chemically related to barbiturates and act to decrease the influx of sodium, thereby decreasing neuronal excitability

c. combination of inhaled and intravenous agents to put someone to sleep

d. lack of sensation

e. major pharmaceutical actions which include analgesia, antipyretic, and antiplatelet

f. pain that is transmitted to other parts of the body via common nerve pathways

g. use of CNS depressants as a premedication before the introduction of anesthesia

h. infusion pumps that provide the patient with the ability to control the amount of analgesia

i. condition in which the patient does not feel pain, but remains conscious

j. fine tremble of the eye when holding a lateral gaze

k. pain receptors in the dermis

l. substances that inhibit the transmission of painful sensations to the brain and spinal cord

m. amount of stimulus required to elicit a pain response

n. difficult movement

o. disequilibria in walk that resembles a drunkard's stagger

CHAPTER **32**

PRINCIPLES OF ELECTROCARDIOGRAPHY

Case Study

Your unit responds to a "heart fluttering" call. Your patient is a 78-year-old woman who complains of her heart "fluttering" in her chest. "I just can't get my breath," she tells you. A quick check of her vital signs reveals the following: pulse is 90 and irregular; BP is 122/74; respirations are 22 and nonlabored. You apply oxygen as your partner applies the cardiac monitor. As the beeps from the monitor start, you hear that the rhythm is irregularly irregular—there seems to be no pattern to the rhythm.

Decision Time

1. What rhythm do you expect?

_____

_____

You load the patient into the ambulance and begin the transport to the local hospital.

2. What intervention is needed for this patient?

_____

_____

While en route to the hospital, you notice that the monitor tracing becomes unclear. You see that one of the patient cables has become detached. You reconnect the cable and return to a clear tracing.

In Retrospect . . .

3. How would treatment have been different if the patient was unstable?

_____

_____

Practice Questions
Multiple Choice

Select the best answer for each of the following questions.

1. Which types of muscle cells have the qualities of excitability and contractability?
   a. cardiac muscle
   b. smooth muscle
   c. striated muscle
   d. all of the above

2. This term refers to the cell's ability to generate its own electrical activity.
   a. automaticity
   b. conductivity
   c. excitability
   d. action potential

3. Which of the following terms describes the ability of cardiac muscle fibers to shorten?
   a. conductivity
   b. excitability
   c. contractility
   d. none of the above

4. Which of the following describes a lead?
   a. wire that connects the ECG monitor to the patient
   b. view of the electrical activity of the heart from a specific vantage point
   c. one of three patient cables
   d. none of the above

5. Which of the following are the standard leads?
   a. I, II, aVL
   b. I, II, III
   c. I, II, aVR
   d. RA, LA, LL

6. Which of the following is represented by Lead II?
   a. the change of voltage between the left arm and the left leg
   b. the change of voltage between the right arm and the left arm
   c. the change of voltage between the right arm and left leg
   d. the change of voltage between the left arm and the right leg

7. Which of the following is represented by Lead I?
   a. the change of voltage between the left arm and the left leg
   b. the change of voltage between the right arm and the left arm
   c. the change of voltage between the right arm and left leg
   d. the change of voltage between the left arm and the right leg

8. Which of the following is represented by Lead III?
   a. the change of voltage between the left arm and the left leg
   b. the change of voltage between the right arm and the left arm
   c. the change of voltage between the right arm and left leg
   d. the change of voltage between the left arm and the right leg

9. Which of the following waveforms on the ECG represents septal depolarization, has a downward or negative deflection, and is the first deflection of the QRS complex?
   a. P wave
   b. Q wave
   c. R wave
   d. S wave

10. Which of the following represents the period of time for the stimulus to travel across the atria and delay at the AV node?
   a. PR interval
   b. ST segment
   c. QT interval
   d. TP segment

11. Which phase of cardiac depolarization begins when the fast sodium channels close and chloride enters the cell?
    a. phase 0
    b. phase 1
    c. phase 2
    d. phase 3

12. Which phase begins with a resting cardiac cell that sees a rapid influx of sodium?
    a. phase 0
    b. phase 1
    c. phase 2
    d. phase 3

13. Which phase is considered the plateau phase?
    a. phase 0
    b. phase 1
    c. phase 2
    d. phase 3

14. Which of the following lies within the mediastinum?
    a. heart
    b. trachea
    c. aorta
    d. all of the above

15. What is the innermost layer of the heart called?
    a. myocardium
    b. endocardium
    c. exocardium
    d. syncytium

Fill in the Blank

Complete each sentence by adding the appropriate word in the provided blanks.

16. The thickest layer of the heart is the _____.

17. The term used to describe the atria at rest is called atrial _____.

18. The _____ _____ are strong cords attached to the papillary muscles that prevent the valves from inverting.

19. The percentage of blood pushed and squeezed out of the heart is called the _____ _____.

20. The primary pacemaker in the heart is called the _____ node.

Matching

Match each term with its corresponding description.

_____ 21. interval   a. innermost layer of the heart

_____ 22. SA node   b. mass of cells that act as a unit

_____ 23. endocardium   c. segment and a wave together

_____ 24. automaticity   d. space between waves

_____ 25. segment   e. sac that covers the heart

_____ 26. epicardium   f. ability to create and conduct its own impulses

_____ 27. refractory   g. outermost layer of the heart

_____ 28. pericardium   h. fires at an intrinsic rate of 60 to 100 per minute

_____ 29. AV junction   i. fires at an intrinsic rate of 40 to 60 per minute

_____ 30. functional syncytium   j. unable to respond to a new stimulus

CHAPTER 33

THE MONITORING ECG

Case Study

You respond to a suburban residence where a 78-year-old female is complaining of chest pain and extreme weakness. You arrive to find her lying on the sofa with very pale and diaphoretic skin. Her pulse rate is approximately 35 to 40; blood pressure is 60 palpable. Before you connect the cardiac monitor, you should be getting an idea about what type of rhythm you will be treating.

Decision Time

1. Is your patient stable?

   _____

   _____

2. Is it possible to have a heart rate of 40 and not be symptomatic?

   _____

   _____

You connect the monitor as your partner provides supplemental oxygen. You run a quick rhythm strip (see Figure 33-1).

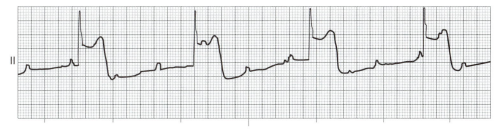

Figure 33-1

3. What is this rhythm?

   _____

   _____

While en route, you start an IV of normal saline and administer 0.5 mg of atropine. A recheck of vital signs reveals a heart rate of 60 and a blood pressure of 100/60.

In Retrospect . . .

4. Your EMT partner asks you to explain a complete heart block. How would you explain it to him?

   _____

   _____

Practice Questions

Fill in the Blank

Complete each sentence by adding the appropriate word in the provided blanks.

1. A process that ensures sweep speed and gain is up to standard is called _____.

2. The stratum _____ is the outermost layer of the epidermis, and does not conduct electricity well.

3. _____ is necessary for the electrode to function.

4. _____ simulates the precordial Lead V1.

5. MCL1 views the _____ wall of the heart.

Matching

Terms

Match each term with its corresponding description.

_____ 6. relative bradycardia

_____ 7. trace

_____ 8. rate counter

_____ 9. pulseless electrical activity

_____ 10. trigeminy

_____ 11. artifact

_____ 12. bigeminy

_____ 13. lead

_____ 14. Lead II

_____ 15. cardiac monitor

_____ 16. equiphasic

_____ 17. morphology

_____ 18. sweep speed

_____ 19. absolute bradycardia

_____ 20. ECG rhythm strip

a. consists of an oscilloscope, and often a printer

b. presence of what is normally a viable rhythm without an accompanying pulse

c. view of the electrical activity of the heart

d. shape

e. negative electrode on right shoulder and positive electrode on left leg

f. 25 mm/second

g. disturbance in the isoelectric line that is a result of outside interference

h. digital readout of the number of ECG complexes that pass in a minute

i. ectopy that occurs every other complex

j. ectopy that occurs every third complex

k. flatline

l. any rate below 60

m. a rate that is too slow for the patient's metabolic needs

n. printed copy of monitor tracing

o. manifestation of left to right movement on the screen

Cardiac Rhythm

Match each term with its corresponding description.

_____ 21. normal sinus rhythm

_____ 22. sinus bradycardia

_____ 23. sinus tachycardia

_____ 24. sinus dysrhythmia

_____ 25. complete heart block

a. no correlation between P waves and QRS complexes

b. regular rhythm with ventricular rate of less than 60

c. regularly irregular rhythm with ventricular rate of 60 to 100

d. regular rhythm with ventricular rate of 60 to 100

e. regular rhythm with ventricular rate of greater than 100

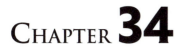

Chapter 34

DIAGNOSTIC ECG— THE 12-LEAD

Case Study

"Time is muscle," says your partner as you pull out of the station en route to a chest pain call. As you ride to the scene, you think about the protocols for acute chest pain. Since you are on a Paramedic unit, you are carrying a 12-lead ECG machine.

Decision Time

1. Why is an early 12-lead ECG important in the care of an acute myocardial infarction (AMI) patient?

_____

_____

2. What information can the 12-lead ECG provide to the Paramedic in the field?

_____

_____

You arrive on the scene to find a 64-year-old woman who complains of pain in her chest wall. You find that the pain increases upon inspiration, and that the patient has had a cough for nearly a week.

3. Do you suspect this pain to be cardiac in nature?

_____

_____

In Retrospect . . .

While this patient is not exhibiting signs of an AMI, you were ready to treat this patient upon arrival.

4. Why is it helpful to think through protocols and possible scenarios on the way to the scene?

_____

_____

Practice Questions
Short Answer

Write a brief answer to each of the following questions.
1. What is the primary advantage to obtaining a 12-lead ECG in the field?

_____

_____

2. What does the Q wave represent?

_____

_____

3. What do inverted T waves represent?

_____

_____

4. What ECG changes might you expect to see associated with hypothermia?

_____

_____

Fill in the Blank

Complete these sentences describing relationship of leads to walls to coronary arteries by adding the appropriate word in the provided blanks.

5. II, III, aVF =   _____   right coronary artery

6. _____ _____ =   anteroseptal   left anterior descending

7. V3, V4 =   _____   left anterior descending

8. V3, V4, V5, V6 =   _____   diagonal

9. I, aVL, V5, V6 =   lateral   _____

10. V1, V2, V3, V4, V5, V6 =   _____   left mainstem

Matching

Electrode Placement

Match each lead name with its corresponding correct electrode placement.

_____ 11. LA   a. 4th right intercostal space at the sternal border

_____ 12. RA   b. right leg over muscle or flesh

_____ 13. LL   c. 4th left intercostal space at the sternal border

_____ 14. RL   d. right arm over muscle or flesh

_____ 15. V1   e. 5th left intercostal space at the midaxillary line

_____ 16. V2   f. left leg over muscle or flesh

_____ 17. V3   g. between V2 and V4

_____ 18. V4   h. 5th left intercostal space at the midclavicular line

_____ 19. V5   i. 5th left intercostal space at the anterior axillary line

_____ 20. V6   j. left arm over muscle or flesh

Terms

Match each term with its corresponding description.

_____ 21. J point

_____ 22. myocardial ischemia

_____ 23. myocardial infarction

_____ 24. situs inversus

_____ 25. transmural ischemia

_____ 26. contiguous leads

_____ 27. pathologic Q wave

_____ 28. necrosis

_____ 29. reverse R wave progression

_____ 30. electrical alternans

a. physiologic process in which dead cells are removed and new cell growth may occur

b. loss of R wave progression suggestive of an anterior wall AMI

c. two or more leads that look at the same wall of the left ventricle

d. myocardial cells are deprived of oxygen and hypoxia ensues

e. amplitude of every other QRS complex varies

f. complete reversal of all thoracoabdominal organs

g. death of myocardial cells

h. marks the start of the ST segment

i. ischemia affecting the entire thickness of the myocardium

j. indicates no depolarization in that portion of the ventricular wall

SECTION **II**

NREMT SKILLS FOR PARAMEDIC CERTIFICATION

1. Patient Assessment—Medical

2. Patient Assessment—Trauma

3. Ventilatory Management
   - Adult
   - Dual Lumen Airway Device (Combitube® or PTL®)

4. Cardiac Management Skills
   - Dynamic Cardiology
   - Static Cardiology

5. IV and Medication Skills
   - Intravenous Therapy
   - Intravenous Bolus Medications

6. Oral Station

7. Pediatric Skills
   - Pediatric (<2 yrs.) Ventilatory Management
   - Pediatric Intraosseous Infusion

8. Random Basic Skills
   - Spinal Immobilization (Seated Patient)
   - Spinal Immobilization (Supine Patient)
   - Bleeding Control/Shock Management

PATIENT ASSESSMENT - MEDICAL

Candidate: _____   Examiner: _____

Date: _____   Signature: _____

Scenario: _____

	Possible Points	Points Awarded
Time Start: _____		
Takes or verbalizes body substance isolation precautions	1	
SCENE SIZE-UP		
Determines the scene/situation is safe	1	
Determines the mechanism of injury/nature of illness	1	
Determines the number of patients	1	
Requests additional help if necessary	1	
Considers stabilization of spine	1	
INITIAL ASSESSMENT		
Verbalizes general impression of the patient	1	
Determines responsiveness/level of consciousness	1	
Determines chief complaint/apparent life-threats	1	
Assesses airway and breathing -Assessment (1 point) -Assures adequate ventilation (1 point) -Initiates appropriate oxygen therapy (1 point)	3	
Assesses circulation -Assesses/controls major bleeding (1 point)　-Assesses skin [either skin color, temperature, or condition] (1 point) -Assesses pulse (1 point)	3	
Identifies priority patients/makes transport decision	1	
FOCUSED HISTORY AND PHYSICAL EXAMINATION/RAPID ASSESSMENT		
History of present illness -Onset (1 point)　　　-Severity (1 point) -Provocation (1 point)　-Time (1 point) -Quality (1 point)　　　-Clarifying questions of associated signs and symptoms as related to OPQRST (2 points) -Radiation (1 point)	8	
Past medical history -Allergies (1 point)　　-Past pertinent history (1 point)　　-Events leading to present illness (1 point) -Medications (1 point)　-Last oral intake (1 point)	5	
Performs focused physical examination [assess affected body part/system or, if indicated, completes rapid assessment] -Cardiovascular　　-Neurological　　　-Integumentary　　　-Reproductive -Pulmonary　　　　-Musculoskeletal　　-GI/GU　　　　　　-Psychological/Social	5	
Vital signs -Pulse (1 point)　　　　　-Respiratory rate and quality (1 point each) -Blood pressure (1 point)　-AVPU (1 point)	5	
Diagnostics [must include application of ECG monitor for dyspnea and chest pain]	2	
States field impression of patient	1	
Verbalizes treatment plan for patient and calls for appropriate intervention(s)	1	
Transport decision re-evaluated	1	
ON-GOING ASSESSMENT		
Repeats initial assessment	1	
Repeats vital signs	1	
Evaluates response to treatments	1	
Repeats focused assessment regarding patient complaint or injuries	1	

Time End: _____

CRITICAL CRITERIA   **TOTAL**   48

_____ Failure to initiate or call for transport of the patient within 15 minute time limit
_____ Failure to take or verbalize body substance isolation precautions
_____ Failure to determine scene safety before approaching patient
_____ Failure to voice and ultimately provide appropriate oxygen therapy
_____ Failure to assess/provide adequate ventilation
_____ Failure to find or appropriately manage problems associated with airway, breathing, hemorrhage or shock [hypoperfusion]
_____ Failure to differentiate patient's need for immediate transportation versus continued assessment and treatment at the scene
_____ Does other detailed or focused history or physical examination before assessing and treating threats to airway, breathing, and circulation
_____ Failure to determine the patient's primary problem
_____ Orders a dangerous or inappropriate intervention
_____ Failure to provide for spinal protection when indicated

You must factually document your rationale for checking any of the above critical items on the reverse side of this form.

p302/8-003k

NREMT Skills for Paramedic Certification   121

PATIENT ASSESSMENT - TRAUMA

Candidate: _____   Examiner: _____

Date: _____   Signature: _____

Scenario # _____

Time Start: _____ NOTE: Areas denoted by "**" may be integrated within sequence of Initial Assessment	Possible Points	Points Awarded
Takes or verbalizes body substance isolation precautions	1	
SCENE SIZE-UP		
Determines the scene/situation is safe	1	
Determines the mechanism of injury/nature of illness	1	
Determines the number of patients	1	
Requests additional help if necessary	1	
Considers stabilization of spine	1	
INITIAL ASSESSMENT/RESUSCITATION		
Verbalizes general impression of the patient	1	
Determines responsiveness/level of consciousness	1	
Determines chief complaint/apparent life-threats	1	
Airway -Opens and assesses airway (1 point) -Inserts adjunct as indicated (1 point)	2	

Breathing
    -Assess breathing (1 point)
    -Assures adequate ventilation (1 point)
    -Initiates appropriate oxygen therapy (1 point)
    -Manages any injury which may compromise breathing/ventilation (1 point)
	4	

Circulation
    -Checks pulse (1point)
    -Assess skin [either skin color, temperature, or condition] (1 point)
    -Assesses for and controls major bleeding if present (1 point)
    -Initiates shock management (1 point)
	4	

Identifies priority patients/makes transport decision	1	
FOCUSED HISTORY AND PHYSICAL EXAMINATION/RAPID TRAUMA ASSESSMENT		
Selects appropriate assessment	1	
Obtains, or directs assistant to obtain, baseline vital signs	1	
Obtains SAMPLE history	1	
DETAILED PHYSICAL EXAMINATION		

Head
    -Inspects mouth**, nose**, and assesses facial area (1 point)
    -Inspects and palpates scalp and ears (1 point)
    -Assesses eyes for PERRL** (1 point)
	3	

Neck**
    -Checks position of trachea (1 point)
    -Checks jugular veins (1 point)
    -Palpates cervical spine (1 point)
	3	

Chest**
    -Inspects chest (1 point)
    -Palpates chest (1 point)
    -Auscultates chest (1 point)
	3	

Abdomen/pelvis**
    -Inspects and palpates abdomen (1 point)
    -Assesses pelvis (1 point)
    -Verbalizes assessment of genitalia/perineum as needed (1 point)
	3	

Lower extremities** -Inspects, palpates, and assesses motor, sensory, and distal circulatory functions (1 point/leg)	2	
Upper extremities -Inspects, palpates, and assesses motor, sensory, and distal circulatory functions (1 point/arm)	2	

Posterior thorax, lumbar, and buttocks**
    -Inspects and palpates posterior thorax (1 point)
    -Inspects and palpates lumbar and buttocks area (1 point)
	2	

Manages secondary injuries and wounds appropriately	1	
Performs ongoing assessment	1	
Time End: _____ **TOTAL**	43	

CRITICAL CRITERIA

_____ Failure to initiate or call for transport of the patient within 10 minute time limit
_____ Failure to take or verbalize body substance isolation precautions
_____ Failure to determine scene safety
_____ Failure to assess for and provide spinal protection when indicated
_____ Failure to voice and ultimately provide high concentration of oxygen
_____ Failure to assess/provide adequate ventilation
_____ Failure to find or appropriately manage problems associated with airway, breathing, hemorrhage or shock [hypoperfusion]
_____ Failure to differentiate patient's need for immediate transportation versus continued assessment/treatment at the scene
_____ Does other detailed/focused history or physical exam before assessing/treating threats to airway, breathing, and circulation
_____ Orders a dangerous or inappropriate intervention

You must factually document your rationale for checking any of the above critical items on the reverse side of this form.

VENTILATORY MANAGEMENT - ADULT

Candidate: _____ Examiner: _____

Date: _____ Signature: _____

NOTE: If candidate elects to ventilate initially with BVM attached to reservoir and oxygen, full credit must be awarded for steps denoted by "**" so long as first ventilation is delivered within 30 seconds.

	Possible Points	Points Awarded
Takes or verbalizes body substance isolation precautions	1	
Opens the airway manually	1	
Elevates tongue, inserts simple adjunct [oropharyngeal or nasopharyngeal airway]	1	
NOTE: Examiner now informs candidate no gag reflex is present and patient accepts adjunct		
**Ventilates patient immediately with bag-valve-mask device unattached to oxygen	1	
**Ventilates patient with room air	1	
NOTE: Examiner now informs candidate that ventilation is being performed without difficulty and that pulse oximetry indicates the patient's blood oxygen saturation is 85%		
Attaches oxygen reservoir to bag-valve-mask device and connects to high flow oxygen regulator [12-15 L/minute]	1	
Ventilates patient at a rate of 10-12/minute with appropriate volumes	1	
NOTE: After 30 seconds, examiner auscultates and reports breath sounds are present, equal bilaterally and medical direction has ordered intubation. The examiner must now take over ventilation.		
Directs assistant to pre-oxygenate patient	1	
Identifies/selects proper equipment for intubation	1	
Checks equipment for: -Cuff leaks (1 point) -Laryngoscope operational with bulb tight (1 point)	2	
NOTE: Examiner to remove OPA and move out of the way when candidate is prepared to intubate		
Positions head properly	1	
Inserts blade while displacing tongue	1	
Elevates mandible with laryngoscope	1	
Introduces ET tube and advances to proper depth	1	
Inflates cuff to proper pressure and disconnects syringe	1	
Directs ventilation of patient	1	
Confirms proper placement by auscultation bilaterally over each lung and over epigastrium	1	
NOTE: Examiner to ask, "If you had proper placement, what should you expect to hear?"		
Secures ET tube [may be verbalized]	1	
NOTE: Examiner now asks candidate, "Please demonstrate one additional method of verifying proper tube placement in this patient."		
Identifies/selects proper equipment	1	
Verbalizes findings and interpretations [compares indicator color to the colorimetric scale or EDD recoil and states findings]	1	
NOTE: Examiner now states, "You see secretions in the tube and hear gurgling sounds with the patient's exhalation."		
Identifies/selects a flexible suction catheter	1	
Pre-oxygenates patient	1	
Marks maximum insertion length with thumb and forefinger	1	
Inserts catheter into the ET tube leaving catheter port open	1	
At proper insertion depth, covers catheter port and applies suction while withdrawing catheter	1	
Ventilates/directs ventilation of patient as catheter is flushed with sterile water	1	
TOTAL	27	

CRITICAL CRITERIA

_____ Failure to initiate ventilations within 30 seconds after applying gloves or interrupts ventilations for greater than 30 seconds at any time
_____ Failure to take or verbalize body substance isolation precautions
_____ Failure to voice and ultimately provide high oxygen concentrations [at least 85%]
_____ Failure to ventilate patient at a rate of 10 - 12 / minute
_____ Failure to provide adequate volumes per breath [maximum 2 errors/minute permissible]
_____ Failure to pre-oxygenate patient prior to intubation and suctioning
_____ Failure to successfully intubate within 3 attempts
_____ Failure to disconnect syringe **immediately** after inflating cuff of ET tube
_____ Uses teeth as a fulcrum
_____ Failure to assure proper tube placement by auscultation bilaterally **and** over the epigastrium
_____ If used, stylette extends beyond end of ET tube
_____ Inserts any adjunct in a manner dangerous to the patient
_____ Suctions the patient for more than 10 seconds
_____ Does not suction the patient

You must factually document your rationale for checking any of the above critical items on the reverse side of this form.

DUAL LUMEN AIRWAY DEVICE (COMBITUBE® OR PTL®)

Candidate: _____ Examiner: _____

Date: _____ Signature: _____

NOTE: If candidate elects to initially ventilate with BVM attached to reservoir and oxygen, full credit must be awarded for steps denoted by "**" so long as first ventilation is delivered within 30 seconds.

	Possible Points	Points Awarded
Takes or verbalizes body substance isolation precautions	1	
Opens the airway manually	1	
Elevates tongue, inserts simple adjunct [oropharyngeal or nasopharyngeal airway]	1	
NOTE: Examiner now informs candidate no gag reflex is present and patient accepts adjunct		
**Ventilates patient immediately with bag-valve-mask device unattached to oxygen	1	
**Hyperventilates patient with room air	1	
NOTE: Examiner now informs candidate that ventilation is being performed without difficulty		
Attaches oxygen reservoir to bag-valve-mask device and connects to high flow oxygen regulator [12-15 L/minute]	1	
Ventilates patient at a rate of 10-12/minute with appropriate volumes	1	
NOTE: After 30 seconds, examiner auscultates and reports breath sounds are present and equal bilaterally and medical control has ordered insertion of a dual lumen airway. The examiner must now take over ventilation.		
Directs assistant to pre-oxygenate patient	1	
Checks/prepares airway device	1	
Lubricates distal tip of the device [may be verbalized]	1	
NOTE: Examiner to remove OPA and move out of the way when candidate is prepared to insert device		
Positions head properly	1	
Performs a tongue-jaw lift	1	

☐ USES COMBITUBE®	☐ USES PTL®	Possible Points	Points Awarded
Inserts device in mid-line and to depth so printed ring is at level of teeth	Inserts device in mid-line until bite block flange is at level of teeth	1	
Inflates pharyngeal cuff with proper volume and removes syringe	Secures strap	1	
Inflates distal cuff with proper volume and removes syringe	Blows into tube #1 to adequately inflate both cuffs	1	
Attaches/directs attachment of BVM to the first [esophageal placement] lumen and ventilates		1	
Confirms placement and ventilation through correct lumen by observing chest rise, auscultation over the epigastrium, and bilaterally over each lung		1	

	Possible Points	Points Awarded
NOTE: The examiner states, "You do not see rise and fall of the chest and you only hear sounds over the epigastrium."		
Attaches/directs attachment of BVM to the second [endotracheal placement] lumen and ventilates	1	
Confirms placement and ventilation through correct lumen by observing chest rise, auscultation over the epigastrium, and bilaterally over each lung	1	
NOTE: The examiner confirms adequate chest rise, absent sounds over the epigastrium, and equal bilateral breath sounds.		
Secures device or confirms that the device remains properly secured	1	
TOTAL	**20**	

CRITICAL CRITERIA

_____ Failure to initiate ventilations within 30 seconds after taking body substance isolation precautions or interrupts ventilations for greater than 30 seconds at any time

_____ Failure to take or verbalize body substance isolation precautions

_____ Failure to voice and ultimately provide high oxygen concentrations [at least 85%]

_____ Failure to ventilate patient at a rate of 10-12/minute

_____ Failure to provide adequate volumes per breath [maximum 2 errors/minute permissible]

_____ Failure to pre-oxygenate patient prior to insertion of the dual lumen airway device

_____ Failure to insert the dual lumen airway device at a proper depth or at either proper place within 3 attempts

_____ Failure to inflate both cuffs properly

_____ **Combitube** - failure to remove the syringe immediately after inflation of each cuff
      PTL - failure to secure the strap prior to cuff inflation

_____ Failure to confirm that the proper lumen of the device is being ventilated by observing chest rise, auscultation over the epigastrium, and bilaterally over each lung

_____ Inserts any adjunct in a manner dangerous to patient

You must factually document your rationale for checking any of the above critical items on the reverse side of this form.

DYNAMIC CARDIOLOGY

Candidate: _____ Examiner: _____

Date: _____ Signature: _____

SET #_____

Level of Testing:　　□ NREMT-Intermediate/99　　　□ NREMT-Paramedic

	Possible Points	Points Awarded
Time Start:_____		
Takes or verbalizes infection control precautions	1	
Checks level of responsiveness	1	
Checks ABCs	1	
Initiates CPR when appropriate [verbally]	1	
Attaches ECG monitor in a timely fashion [patches, pads or paddles]	1	
Correctly interprets initial rhythm	1	
Appropriately manages initial rhythm	2	
Notes change in rhythm	1	
Checks patient condition to include pulse and, if appropriate, BP	1	
Correctly interprets second rhythm	1	
Appropriately manages second rhythm	2	
Notes change in rhythm	1	
Checks patient condition to include pulse and, if appropriate, BP	1	
Correctly interprets third rhythm	1	
Appropriately manages third rhythm	2	
Notes change in rhythm	1	
Checks patient condition to include pulse and, if appropriate, BP	1	
Correctly interprets fourth rhythm	1	
Appropriately manages fourth rhythm	2	
Orders high percentages of supplemental oxygen at proper times	1	
Time End: _____　　　　　　　　　　TOTAL	24	

CRITICAL CRITERIA

_____ Failure to deliver any shock in a timely manner

_____ Failure to verify rhythm before delivering each shock

_____ Failure to ensure the safety of self and others [verbalizes "All clear" and observes]

_____ Inability to deliver DC shock [does not use machine properly]

_____ Failure to demonstrate acceptable shock sequence

_____ Failure to immediately order initiation or resumption of CPR when appropriate

_____ Failure to order correct management of airway [ET when appropriate]

_____ Failure to order administration of appropriate oxygen at proper time

_____ Failure to diagnose or treat 2 or more rhythms correctly

_____ Orders administration of an inappropriate drug or lethal dosage

_____ Failure to correctly diagnose or adequately treat v-fib, v-tach, or asystole

You must factually document your rationale for checking any of the above critical items on the reverse side of this form.

p306/8-003k

National Registry of Emergency Medical Technicians
Advanced Level Practical Examination

STATIC CARDIOLOGY

Candidate: _____ Examiner: _____

Date: _____ Signature: _____

SET #_____

Level of Testing: ☐ NREMT-Intermediate/99   ☐ NREMT-Paramedic

Note: No points for treatment may be awarded if the diagnosis is incorrect.
   Only document incorrect responses in spaces provided.

Time Start:_____

	Possible Points	Points Awarded
STRIP #1		
Diagnosis:	1	
Treatment:	2	
STRIP #2		
Diagnosis:	1	
Treatment:	2	
STRIP #3		
Diagnosis:	1	
Treatment:	2	
STRIP #4		
Diagnosis:	1	
Treatment:	2	
Time End: _____ **TOTAL**	12	

© 2000 National Registry of Emergency Medical Technicians, Inc., Columbus, OH
All materials subject to this copyright may be photocopied for the non-commercial purpose of educational or scientific advancement.

p307/8-003k

126   Foundations of Paramedic Care Study Guide

© 2010 Cengage Learning. All Rights Reserved. May not be scanned, copied or duplicated, or posted to a publicly accessible website, in whole or in part.

INTRAVENOUS THERAPY

Candidate: _____ Examiner: _____

Date: _____ Signature: _____

Level of Testing: ❑ NREMT-Intermediate/85   ❑ NREMT-Intermediate/99   ❑ NREMT-Paramedic

Time Start: _____

	Possible Points	Points Awarded
Checks selected IV fluid for: -Proper fluid (1 point) -Clarity (1 point)	2	
Selects appropriate catheter	1	
Selects proper administration set	1	
Connects IV tubing to the IV bag	1	
Prepares administration set [fills drip chamber and flushes tubing]	1	
Cuts or tears tape [at any time before venipuncture]	1	
Takes/verbalizes body substance isolation precautions [prior to venipuncture]	1	
Applies tourniquet	1	
Palpates suitable vein	1	
Cleanses site appropriately	1	
Performs venipuncture -Inserts stylette (1 point) -Notes or verbalizes flashback (1 point) -Occludes vein proximal to catheter (1 point) -Removes stylette (1 point) -Connects IV tubing to catheter (1 point)	5	
Disposes/verbalizes disposal of needle in proper container	1	
Releases tourniquet	1	
Runs IV for a brief period to assure patent line	1	
Secures catheter [tapes securely or verbalizes]	1	
Adjusts flow rate as appropriate	1	

Time End: _____   **TOTAL** 21

CRITICAL CRITERIA

____ Failure to establish a patent and properly adjusted IV within 6 minute time limit
____ Failure to take or verbalize body substance isolation precautions prior to performing venipuncture
____ Contaminates equipment or site without appropriately correcting situation
____ Performs any improper technique resulting in the potential for uncontrolled hemorrhage, catheter shear, or air embolism
____ Failure to successfully establish IV within 3 attempts during 6 minute time limit
____ Failure to dispose/verbalize disposal of needle in proper container

NOTE: Check here (_____) if candidate did not establish a patent IV and do not evaluate IV Bolus Medications.

INTRAVENOUS BOLUS MEDICATIONS

Time Start: _____

	Possible Points	Points Awarded
Asks patient for known allergies	1	
Selects correct medication	1	
Assures correct concentration of drug	1	
Assembles prefilled syringe correctly and dispels air	1	
Continues body substance isolation precautions	1	
Cleanses injection site [Y-port or hub]	1	
Reaffirms medication	1	
Stops IV flow [pinches tubing or shuts off]	1	
Administers correct dose at proper push rate	1	
Disposes/verbalizes proper disposal of syringe and needle in proper container	1	
Flushes tubing [runs wide open for a brief period]	1	
Adjusts drip rate to TKO/KVO	1	
Verbalizes need to observe patient for desired effect/adverse side effects	1	

Time End: _____   **TOTAL** 13

CRITICAL CRITERIA

____ Failure to begin administration of medication within 3 minute time limit
____ Contaminates equipment or site without appropriately correcting situation
____ Failure to adequately dispel air resulting in potential for air embolism
____ Injects improper drug or dosage [wrong drug, incorrect amount, or pushes at inappropriate rate]
____ Failure to flush IV tubing after injecting medication
____ Recaps needle or failure to dispose/verbalize disposal of syringe and needle in proper container

You must factually document your rationale for checking any of the above critical items on the reverse side of this form.

p309/8-003k

National Registry of Emergency Medical Technicians
Advanced Level Practical Examination
ORAL STATION

Candidate: _____ Examiner: _____

Date: _____ Signature: _____

Scenario: _____

Time Start: _____

	Possible Points	Points Awarded
Scene Management		
Thoroughly assessed and took deliberate actions to control the scene	3	
Assessed the scene, identified potential hazards, did not put anyone in danger	2	
Incompletely assessed or managed the scene	1	
Did not assess or manage the scene	0	
Patient Assessment		
Completed an organized assessment and integrated findings to expand further assessment	3	
Completed initial, focused, and ongoing assessments	2	
Performed an incomplete or disorganized assessment	1	
Did not complete an initial assessment	0	
Patient Management		
Managed all aspects of the patient's condition and anticipated further needs	3	
Appropriately managed the patient's presenting condition	2	
Performed an incomplete or disorganized management	1	
Did not manage life-threatening conditions	0	
Interpersonal relations		
Established rapport and interacted in an organized, therapeutic manner	3	
Interacted and responded appropriately with patient, crew, and bystanders	2	
Used inappropriate communication techniques	1	
Demonstrated intolerance for patient, bystanders, and crew	0	
Integration (verbal report, field impression, and transport decision)		
Stated correct field impression and pathophysiological basis, provided succinct and accurate verbal report including social/psychological concerns, and considered alternate transport destinations	3	
Stated correct field impression, provided succinct and accurate verbal report, and appropriately stated transport decision	2	
Stated correct field impression, provided inappropriate verbal report or transport decision	1	
Stated incorrect field impression or did not provide verbal report	0	

Time End: _____ **TOTAL** | 15 | |

Critical Criteria

_____ Failure to appropriately address any of the scenario's "Mandatory Actions"

_____ Performs or orders any harmful or dangerous action or intervention

You must factually document your rationale for checking any of the above critical items on the reverse side of this form.

p308/8-003k

PEDIATRIC (<2 yrs.) VENTILATORY MANAGEMENT

Candidate: _____   Examiner _____

Date: _____   Signature: _____

NOTE: If candidate elects to ventilate initially with BVM attached to reservoir and oxygen, full credit must be awarded for steps denoted by "***" so long as first ventilation is delivered within 30 seconds.

	Possible Points	Points Awarded
Takes or verbalizes body substance isolation precautions	1	
Opens the airway manually	1	
Elevates tongue, inserts simple adjunct [oropharyngeal or nasopharyngeal airway]	1	
NOTE: Examiner now informs candidate no gag reflex is present and patient accepts adjunct		
**Ventilates patient immediately with bag-valve-mask device unattached to oxygen	1	
**Ventilates patient with room air	1	
NOTE: Examiner now informs candidate that ventilation is being performed without difficulty and that pulse oximetry indicates the patient's blood oxygen saturation is 85%		
Attaches oxygen reservoir to bag-valve-mask device and connects to high flow oxygen regulator [12-15 L/minute]	1	
Ventilates patient at a rate of 12-20/minute and assures visible chest rise	1	
NOTE: After 30 seconds, examiner auscultates and reports breath sounds are present, equal bilaterally and medical direction has ordered intubation. The examiner must now take over ventilation.		
Directs assistant to pre-oxygenate patient	1	
Identifies/selects proper equipment for intubation	1	
Checks laryngoscope to assure operational with bulb tight	1	
NOTE: Examiner to remove OPA and move out of the way when candidate is prepared to intubate		
Places patient in neutral or sniffing position	1	
Inserts blade while displacing tongue	1	
Elevates mandible with laryngoscope	1	
Introduces ET tube and advances to proper depth	1	
Directs ventilation of patient	1	
Confirms proper placement by auscultation bilaterally over each lung and over epigastrium	1	
NOTE: Examiner to ask, "If you had proper placement, what should you expect to hear?"		
Secures ET tube [may be verbalized]	1	

TOTAL   17

CRITICAL CRITERIA

_____ Failure to initiate ventilations within 30 seconds after applying gloves or interrupts ventilations for greater than 30 seconds at any time

_____ Failure to take or verbalize body substance isolation precautions

_____ Failure to pad under the torso to allow neutral head position or sniffing position

_____ Failure to voice and ultimately provide high oxygen concentrations [at least 85%]

_____ Failure to ventilate patient at a rate of 12-20/minute

_____ Failure to provide adequate volumes per breath [maximum 2 errors/minute permissible]

_____ Failure to pre-oxygenate patient prior to intubation

_____ Failure to successfully intubate within 3 attempts

_____ Uses gums as a fulcrum

_____ Failure to assure proper tube placement by auscultation bilaterally **and** over the epigastrium

_____ Inserts any adjunct in a manner dangerous to the patient

_____ Attempts to use any equipment not appropriate for the pediatric patient

You must factually document your rationale for checking any of the above critical items on the reverse side of this form.

p305/8-003k

National Registry of Emergency Medical Technicians
Advanced Level Practical Examination

PEDIATRIC INTRAOSSEOUS INFUSION

Candidate: _____   Examiner: _____

Date: _____   Signature: _____

Time Start:_____

	Possible Points	Points Awarded
Checks selected IV fluid for: -Proper fluid (1 point) -Clarity (1 point)	2	
Selects appropriate equipment to include: -IO needle (1 point) -Syringe (1 point) -Saline (1 point) -Extension set (1 point)	4	
Selects proper administration set	1	
Connects administration set to bag	1	
Prepares administration set [fills drip chamber and flushes tubing]	1	
Prepares syringe and extension tubing	1	
Cuts or tears tape [at any time before IO puncture]	1	
Takes or verbalizes body substance isolation precautions [prior to IO puncture]	1	
Identifies proper anatomical site for IO puncture	1	
Cleanses site appropriately	1	
Performs IO puncture: -Stabilizes tibia (1 point) -Inserts needle at proper angle (1 point) -Advances needle with twisting motion until "pop" is felt (1 point) -Unscrews cap and removes stylette from needle (1 point)	4	
Disposes of needle in proper container	1	
Attaches administration set to IO needle (with or without 3-way)	1	
Slowly injects saline to assure proper placement of needle	1	
Adjusts flow rate as appropriate	1	
Secures needle with tape and supports with bulky dressing	1	

Time End: _____   **TOTAL**   23

CRITICAL CRITERIA

_____ Failure to establish a patent and properly adjusted IO line within the 6 minute time limit
_____ Failure to take or verbalize body substance isolation precautions prior to performing IO puncture
_____ Contaminates equipment or site without appropriately correcting situation
_____ Performs any improper technique resulting in the potential for air embolism
_____ Failure to assure correct needle placement
_____ Failure to successfully establish IO infusion within 2 attempts during 6 minute time limit
_____ Performing IO puncture in an unacceptable manner [improper site, incorrect needle angle, etc.]
_____ Failure to dispose of needle in proper container
_____ Orders or performs any dangerous or potentially harmful procedure

You must factually document your rationale for checking any of the above critical items on the reverse side of this form.

p310/8-003k

SPINAL IMMOBILIZATION (SEATED PATIENT)

Candidate: _____ Examiner: _____

Date: _____ Signature: _____

	Possible Points	Points Awarded
Time Start: _____		
Takes or verbalizes body substance isolation precautions	1	
Directs assistant to place/maintain head in the neutral, in-line position	1	
Directs assistant to maintain manual immobilization of the head	1	
Reassesses motor, sensory, and circulatory function in each extremity	1	
Applies appropriately sized extrication collar	1	
Positions the immobilization device behind the patient	1	
Secures the device to the patient's torso	1	
Evaluates torso fixation and adjusts as necessary	1	
Evaluates and pads behind the patient's head as necessary	1	
Secures the patient's head to the device	1	
Verbalizes moving the patient to a long backboard	1	
Reassesses motor, sensory, and circulatory function in each extremity	1	
Time End: _____ **TOTAL**	12	

CRITICAL CRITERIA

_____ Did not immediately direct or take manual immobilization of the head

_____ Did not properly apply appropriately sized cervical collar before ordering release of manual immobilization

_____ Released or ordered release of manual immobilization before it was maintained mechanically

_____ Manipulated or moved patient excessively causing potential spinal compromise

_____ Head immobilized to the device **before** device sufficiently secured to torso

_____ Device moves excessively up, down, left, or right on the patient's torso

_____ Head immobilization allows for excessive movement

_____ Torso fixation inhibits chest rise, resulting in respiratory compromise

_____ Upon completion of immobilization, head is not in a neutral, in-line position

_____ Did not reassess motor, sensory, and circulatory functions in each extremity after voicing immobilization to the long backboard

You must factually document your rationale for checking any of the above critical items on the reverse side of this form.

p311/8-003k

National Registry of Emergency Medical Technicians
Advanced Level Practical Examination

SPINAL IMMOBILIZATION (SUPINE PATIENT)

Candidate:_____ Examiner:_____

Date: _____ Signature:_____

Time Start: _____	Possible Points	Points Awarded
Takes or verbalizes body substance isolation precautions	1	
Directs assistant to place/maintain head in the neutral, in-line position	1	
Directs assistant to maintain manual immobilization of the head	1	
Reassesses motor, sensory, and circulatory function in each extremity	1	
Applies appropriately sized extrication collar	1	
Positions the immobilization device appropriately	1	
Directs movement of the patient onto the device without compromising the integrity of the spine	1	
Applies padding to voids between the torso and the device as necessary	1	
Immobilizes the patient's torso to the device	1	
Evaluates and pads behind the patient's head as necessary	1	
Immobilizes the patient's head to the device	1	
Secures the patient's legs to the device	1	
Secures the patient's arms to the device	1	
Reassesses motor, sensory, and circulatory function in each extremity	1	

Time End: _____   **TOTAL**   14

CRITICAL CRITERIA

_____ Did not immediately direct or take manual immobilization of the head
_____ Did not properly apply appropriately sized cervical collar before ordering release of manual immobilization
_____ Released or ordered release of manual immobilization before it was maintained mechanically
_____ Manipulated or moved patient excessively causing potential spinal compromise
_____ Head immobilized to the device **before** device sufficiently secured to torso
_____ Patient moves excessively up, down, left, or right on the device
_____ Head immobilization allows for excessive movement
_____ Upon completion of immobilization, head is not in a neutral, in-line position
_____ Did not reassess motor, sensory, and circulatory functions in each extremity after voicing immobilization to the device

You must factually document your rationale for checking any of the above critical items on the reverse side of this form.

BLEEDING CONTROL/SHOCK MANAGEMENT

Candidate: _____ Examiner: _____

Date: _____ Signature: _____

	Possible Points	Points Awarded
Time Start:_____		
Takes or verbalizes body substance isolation precautions	1	
Applies direct pressure to the wound	1	
NOTE: The examiner must now inform the candidate that the wound continues to bleed.		
Applies tourniquet	1	
NOTE: The examiner must now inform the candidate that the patient is exhibiting signs and symptoms of hypoperfusion.		
Properly positions the patient	1	
Administers high concentration oxygen	1	
Initiates steps to prevent heat loss from the patient	1	
Indicates the need for immediate transportation	1	
Time End: _____ **TOTAL**	7	

CRITICAL CRITERIA

_____ Did not take or verbalize body substance isolation precautions

_____ Did not apply high concentration of oxygen

_____ Did not control hemorrhage using correct procedures in a timely manner

_____ Did not indicate the need for immediate transportation

You must factually document your rationale for checking any of the above critical items on the reverse side of this form.

p313/8-003k

SECTION III

ANSWERS
TO QUESTIONS

Chapter 1

Case Study #1

1. The answer will depend on the student's personal response. Each answer is as unique as each individual, but should include what motivated the student to study paramedicine.

Case Study #2

1. Paramedics should realize that because they operate under the medical license of a physician or medical authority (varies by state), they are responsible to the physician in assuring quality patient care.

2. The traits of a profession include:
   - extensive educational preparation
   - accreditation of educational programs
   - mentoring
   - certification
   - licensing
   - professional development
   - professional societies
   - code of ethics

3. By acting under the physician's license, the Paramedic is acting as a steward of that license. As a steward, the Paramedic takes great care in protecting the integrity of the license.

4. Since there are not enough physicians available to provide out-of-hospital emergency care, Dr. Houston and physicians like him entrust certified and licensed Paramedics who have extensive educational preparation to provide care for the sick and injured.

Practice Questions

Multiple Choice

1. d
2. c
3. a
4. b
5. d

Short Answer

6. Paramedics are leaders not by virtue of their position, but by their ability to affect the behavior of other members of the team to accomplish the goal of patient care.

7. In the past, Paramedics were considered auxiliary healthcare providers—unlicensed providers who received much of their training on the job—and were not considered to be healthcare professionals. Today, an increasing number of Paramedics graduate from postsecondary educational institutions—many of which are accredited by an external entity.

8. The traits of a profession include:
   - extensive educational preparation
   - accreditation of educational programs
   - mentoring
   - certification
   - licensing
   - professional development
   - professional societies
   - code of ethics

9. A national examination would help Paramedics to transfer from one geographical area to another by assuring a common entry point into the profession.

10. The National Registry of EMTs provides a certification of practical testing and written examinations for Paramedic certification.

11. The National Association of EMTs speaks on behalf of Paramedics.

12. These two reports, released in 2006, spoke of the dysfunctional and fragmented emergency services in the United States.

13. The mnemonic PEARLS stands for partnership, empathy, apology, respect, legitimization, and support.

14. Empathy is seeking to understand how the patient feels by putting oneself in his shoes. Sympathy is actually suffering with the patient. The Paramedic should strive to understand the patient's feelings (empathize) without feeling the patient's feelings (sympathize).

Fill in the Blank

15. professional development
16. medical practice act
17. shared practice
18. steward
19. continuous quality improvement
20. followership

21. research
22. certification (Licensure would also be an appropriate answer depending upon the state.)
23. respect
24. legitimization
25. code, ethics

Chapter 2
Case Study

1. You can use your Paramedic textbook, the Internet, or a library to locate reference material for your presentation.

2. The answer will depend on the student's personal response. There is no right or wrong answer.

3. The TV show *Emergency!* was about the establishment of the Paramedic program in L.A. County.

4. The answer will depend on the student's personal response. There is no right or wrong answer.

5. The answer will depend on the student's personal response. There is no right or wrong answer.

6. Paramedics and physicians could tell you about the history of the local EMS system.

Practice Questions
Multiple Choice

1. c
2. a
3. c
4. b
5. d
6. b
7. c
8. d

9. d
10. d
11. a
12. b
13. d
14. c
15. a

Short Answer

16. EMS became recognized as part of the public health services in the 1960s.

17. The National EMS Core Content lists the knowledge and skills necessary to provide emergency care.

18. There are four levels of EMS providers delineated by the National EMS Scope of Practice.

19. A state-issued license gives the holder the right to perform a function.

20. Certification takes place in EMS upon completion of a specific educational program.

Fill in the Blank

21. fixed post

22. event driven

23. Specialty Care Transport

24. medical oversight

25. direction

26. protocols

27. algorithm

Matching

28. c

29. a

30. b

Chapter 3

Case Study #1

1. Before taking any action, you should consider your personal safety.

2. As part of personal safety, you should take the time to dress appropriately.

3. Since it was a motor vehicle collision with active extrication efforts at the scene, you should have practiced body substance isolation, including eye and face protection due to the potential for flying glass and debris.

4. Since blood was splattered on your face, first wash the blood from your face and eyes. Then, report the potential exposure to your designated infection control officer for appropriate follow-up.

5. To prevent a reoccurrence of this situation, think safety at every point during the call and take appropriate precautions.

Case Study #2

1. The best option is usually retreat, although in this circumstance retreating back to the ambulance might mean running face-to-face into the gunman.

2. The next best option is to take cover—to place a solid object that cannot be penetrated by a projectile between you and the threat.

3. If you had not waited for law enforcement to arrive and secure the scene, you could have arrived in the middle of an altercation.

4. To prevent the chances of being caught in an altercation, you should be preceded by law enforcement in any domestic disturbance call. In addition, if you arrive at a scene and find potential hazards, you should assure that the scene is secure before entering.

Practice Questions

Multiple Choice

1. c

2. a

3. c

4. c

5. d

6. d

7. a

8. b

9. c

10. b

Short Answer

11. Standard immunizations in most EMS agencies are tetanus, diptheria, polio, hepatitis B, and MMR (measles, mumps, and rubella).

12. By taking personal immunizations as part of a plan for personal wellness, the Paramedic will protect himself, his family, and his patients.

13. BSI is a philosophy of infection control in which the Paramedic protects herself from any and all body substances. This is accomplished by wearing gloves along with any other personal protective equipment (PPE) that is warranted for the situation.

14. Taking cover behind a heavy door, vehicle, or some other substantial object is preferred over concealment behind some object that provides less protection.

15. Wellness includes several components, including exercise, eating right, getting enough sleep, being immunized, having interests outside of work, and others, that allow the Paramedic to stay healthy and well. Wellness involves social, spiritual, intellectual, emotional, and physical well-being and a balanced lifestyle.

Fill in the Blank

16. wellness
17. obesity
18. 100
19. education
20. four
21. smoking
22. obesity
23. risk management
24. home
25. initial response
26. due regard
27. personal safety
28. officer-in-charge
29. deadly weapons
30. dangerous instrument

Chapter 4
Case Study

1. The answer will depend on the student's personal response. There is no right or wrong answer.

2. The first step in conducting a research study is to conduct a literature review.

3. Resources available for a literature review include MEDLINE, PubMed, ERIC, local libraries, and local medical schools. A research librarian can also be very helpful in guiding your search.

4. Before conducting research on human subjects, you must get approval from your Institutional Review Board, or IRB.

5. A negative result is just as important as an affirmative result because it is just as important to know that the answer to a research question is "no" as it is to know that the answer is "yes."

Practice Questions
Multiple Choice

1. b
2. c
3. a
4. b
5. c
6. d
7. a
8. a
9. c
10. a

Short Answer

11. The purpose of scientific EMS research is to establish practice that is defendable.

12. Paramedic practices, protocols, and procedures originated from anecdotal experience.

13. A major advantage of evidence-based practice is more cost-effective practices.

14. The most common type of research found in EMS literature is retrospective studies.

15. The strongest type of research is prospective research.

16. The three basic types of research are descriptive studies, observational studies, and experimental studies.

17. The National Research Act of 1974 outlines three principles that address ethical concerns of scientific research: (1) informing participants in a study about participating; (2) eliminating problems of diminished autonomy or the ability to consent; and (3) maintaining justice for participants.

18. In the absence of research, best practices can serve as a guide in determining the best method or most effective way of providing patient care.

19. A type I error in experimental research is a false positive.

20. A type II error in experimental research is a false negative.

21. By conducting research, the Paramedic can provide care that is proven effective.

22. The first step to transform a practice to evidence-based practice is a review of the literature.

23. Peer-reviewed journals provide a critical analysis that provides readers with a degree of confidence that what they are reading meets the profession's standards and is a scholarly work.

Matching

24. c

25. d

26. f

27. b

28. e

29. g

30. a

Chapter 5

Case Study

1. At this point, your first priority should be the care of your patient. An appropriate response would be to assure your patient that you will take her to the hospital and that the bill can be taken care of later.

2. This answer will depend on the student's personal response.

3. This answer will depend on the student's personal response.

4. Yes, you should report this incident to your supervisor.

5. Yes, you should tell your supervisor about your partner's actions.

6. This answer will depend on the student's personal answer.

Practice Questions

Multiple Choice

1. c

2. d

3. a

4. d

5. c

Fill in the Blank

6. system

7. cultural, religious

8. conduct

9. teleological

10. harm

11. duty

12. human

13. moral

14. autonomy

15. veracity

Matching

16. d
17. f
18. e
19. c
20. g

21. h
22. i
23. j
24. b
25. k

Chapter 6

Case Study

1. You should seek informed consent from the patient.

2. If the patient refuses treatment, you do have options. Although you cannot make him seek treatment, the law enforcement officer may place him in custody and allow you to treat and transport him.

3. The mnemonic BARNACLE (**B**enefits, **A**lternatives, **R**isks, **N**ature of procedure, **A**nswers to questions, **C**onsent may be withdrawn, reasonable circumstances if they **L**ack the treatment, **E**xplanations offered in terms the patient could understand) can help you verify you have completed all the necessary steps in acquiring informed consent.

4. Since a 15-year-old has not reached the age of majority, he would not be able to provide consent.

Practice Questions

Multiple Choice

1. b
2. b
3. a
4. d
5. a

6. c
7. d
8. b
9. a
10. c

Short Answer

11. To assure you have completed all the necessary steps for acquiring informed consent, you may use the mnemonic BARNACLE (**B**enefits, **A**lternatives, **R**isks, **N**ature of procedure, **A**nswers to questions, **C**onsent may be withdrawn, reasonable circumstances if they **L**ack the treatment, **E**xplanations offered in terms the patient could understand).

12. Advanced directives are wishes of the patient which are determined in advance, whereas against medical advice (AMA) is refusal of treatment at the time of the treatment.

13. The four core principles are:
    1. Competent people can refuse medical treatment, even at their own peril.
    2. Interests of the state are subordinate to the will of a competent patient.
    3. Healthcare decisions are better made by a physician and the patient than by the court system.
    4. If the patient lacks the ability to make decisions, the patient may assign a surrogate decision maker in her stead.

14. Patient information may be shared only with those who have a legitimate need to know.

15. By referring to previous cases, the judge may assure that the same principles are applied today as they were previously in similar cases.

Matching

16. k
17. j
18. o
19. g
20. n
21. h
22. l
23. d

24. m
25. f
26. b
27. i
28. c
29. a
30. e

Chapter 7

Case Study

1. You should treat this patient like any other with flu-like symptoms and protect yourself with body substance isolation and respiratory precautions. Whether he has the swine flu or a common cold, you don't want to catch it.

2. The local health department should be notified if a reportable communicable disease is suspected.

3. If the patient had swine flu, you should have placed a surgical mask on the patient since he is not in an isolation area.

Practice Questions

Fill in the Blank

1. communities
2. healthcare providers, organizations
3. epidemiology
4. environmental health
5. behavioral
6. occupational
7. predictable
8. nurses
9. public health
10. workplace

11. prevention
12. response
13. quarantine
14. pandemics
15. United Nations
16. malaria
17. workforce
18. physician
19. public health
20. eight

Matching

21. c
22. d
23. a

24. b
25. e

Chapter 8

Case Study

1. Yes, this is most definitely a teaching moment. Since you have the attention of both the injured boy and his friends, this is an excellent time to share the importance of wearing personal protective equipment.

2. Although you could "fuss" at the teenagers, it is unlikely that nagging or stern warnings will be effective. The most effective method may be to share your concern about their safety. By sharing your concern and not being judgmental, you may get the teenagers to listen.

3. This answer will depend on the student's personal response, but it is expected that you can.

4. This injury program utilizes vertical equity.

5. Yes, this program would be an excellent partnership with a local civic organization to provide helmets and pads, as well as a safe place to skate, to those in need.

Practice Questions
Fill in the Blank

1. detection
2. accurate
3. Trauma
4. health
5. nonlethal
6. contained
7. engineering
8. education
9. enforcement
10. economic
11. equity
12. horizontal equity
13. vertical equity
14. teachable moment
15. outcomes evaluation

Matching

16. e
17. d
18. g
19. j
20. a
21. c
22. f
23. b
24. h
25. i

Chapter 9
Case Study

1. This patient is in the acceptance stage of dying.

2. The patient's daughter is most likely in the denial stage.

3. No, you should not insist the patient go to the hospital, although you should offer to take her to the hospital if she desires.

4. No, grief counseling is not among your duties. However, you should offer to refer the patient to a social worker for grief counseling for her family. It is likely that a local hospice agency will provide these services.

5. To better utilize this knowledge, you can check with local hospice and social service agencies to see if your agency can refer patients to them. They may also offer professional development opportunities that you may take to develop your skills.

Practice Questions
Multiple Choice

1. b
2. d
3. c
4. c
5. a
6. d
7. a
8. c
9. a
10. d
11. b
12. c
13. b
14. c
15. a

Matching

16. f

17. b

18. d

19. g

20. c

21. e

22. a

23. j

24. i

25. h

26. l

27. m

28. o

29. k

30. n

Chapter 10

Case Study

1. Stress is causing these symptoms.

2. The sympathetic nervous system is the division of the autonomic nervous system dominating in this case.

3. Norepinephrine, or adrenaline, is the chemical mediator causing these symptoms.

4. If the body has decreased blood flow due to cardiovascular damage, shock, trauma, or other injuries or illnesses, the sympathetic nervous system can help assure the body maintains adequate blood flow.

Practice Questions

Fill in the Blank

1. alarm

2. resistance

3. exhaustion

4. eustress

5. synapse

6. sympathetic

7. parasympathetic

8. heart

9. Alpha$_2$

10. hypertrophy

Matching

11. i

12. f

13. k

14. g

15. d

16. a

17. c

18. j

19. r

20. n

21. q

22. m

23. p

24. h

25. t

26. o

27. e

28. b

29. s

30. l

Chapter 11

Case Study

1. The patient is suffering from hypovolemic shock.

2. The patient is in compensated shock.

3. The treatment should include checking the ABCs, controlling bleeding, providing supplemental oxygen, assuring adequate ventilation, and starting IV of crystalloid or colloid solution.

4. An advantage of starting the IV while en route is faster access to definitive care. A disadvantage is that it is more difficult to start an IV while en route to definitive care.

5. The patient's vital signs improved because bleeding was controlled, supplemental oxygen was provided, and fluid replacement helped improve the patient's circulation of oxygenated blood.

Practice Questions

Multiple Choice

1. a
2. c
3. d
4. b
5. b

6. b
7. c
8. d
9. c
10. a

Fill in the Blank

11. ischemia
12. toxin
13. trauma

14. electroporation
15. barotrauma

Matching

16. n
17. h
18. a
19. e
20. c
21. m
22. f
23. g

24. o
25. j
26. i
27. d
28. l
29. k
30. b

Chapter 12

Case Study

1. The answer will depend on the student's personal response, but might include something like this: Medical terminology is helpful when using that terminology makes your story clearer to a medical professional than using lay terminology. For instance, "right upper quadrant" is more descriptive than "the area just below the right ribs." Medical terminology should make it easier to communicate with other medical professionals.

2. You should not use medical terminology when speaking to a patient or family member. The reason we have the language of medicine is to make the message clearer to others who speak the language. Consequently, you would not speak medicalese to those who do not know the language.

3. Although that sounds like a simple solution, we need the language of medicine so that healthcare professionals can describe things in more detail than is possible in plain English. For instance, "paroxysmal supraventricular tachycardia" (PSVT) is more descriptive and easier for the medical professional to understand than "a sudden occurrence of a fast heart rate of 160 or greater that originates above the ventricles." Medical terminology is an important skill to learn.

Practice Questions

Short Answer

1. As a healthcare professional, the Paramedic should speak the language of medicine.

2. To read medical terms with prefixes and suffixes, one should read the suffix first, then the prefix and root. Think of the way your name is likely listed on the rolls of your Paramedic course: last name, first name, middle name. Use this concept to help you to better interpret medical terms.

3. No, you should use common lay terms when speaking to patients and their families.

4. Do not guess at the meaning of a term. Either look the term up or use the common lay-terminology.

5. It is sometimes necessary to spell out medical terms for clarity.

Matching

Root Words

6. f
7. c
8. j
9. e
10. b
11. h
12. g
13. a
14. d
15. i

Prefixes

16. a
17. b
18. i
19. d
20. g

21. h
22. j
23. e
24. c
25. f

Suffixes

26. i
27. h
28. a
29. c
30. f
31. d
32. e
33. b
34. g
35. j

Chapter 13

Case Study

1. The first priority should be scene safety.

2. The patient's level of consciousness on the AVPU scale is unresponsive.

3. The next step is opening the airway with the head-tilt, chin-lift method and assessing for breathing.

4. You should maintain an open airway and assist ventilations using a bag-valve-mask.

5. The assessment will continue en route.

6. No, you conducted the initial assessment on scene, found the patient to be critical, and transported without delay. By continuing your assessment en route, you got this patient to definitive care in the fastest possible manner while assuring that he was properly ventilated and oxygenated.

Practice Questions
Fill in the Blank

1. primary assessment
2. high
3. low
4. barrier
5. general impression
6. voice, or verbal
7. unresponsive
8. alert, oriented
9. sternal
10. look, listen, feel
11. flail segment
12. 10, 30
13. baseline
14. serial
15. unresponsive

Matching

16. e
17. h
18. d
19. b
20. j
21. f
22. i
23. g
24. a
25. c

Chapter 14
Case Study

1. Yes, you should consider the fear that your patient is likely to have and adjust your approach accordingly.
2. This is considered a person's personal space.
3. The study of nonverbal behavior is called kinesics.
4. She would have likely been afraid and would have withdrawn in distrust.

Practice Questions
Fill in the Blank

1. sent, received
2. communications
3. medical
4. touch
5. open, close
6. why
7. false
8. blocking
9. clarification, summarizing
10. cultural competence

Matching

11. j
12. f
13. o
14. n
15. k
16. a
17. g
18. b
19. i
20. h
21. d
22. m
23. l
24. e
25. c

Chapter 15

Case Study

1. The mnemonic OPQRST AS/PN is most appropriate to assess the patient's present illness.

2. The mnemonic SAMPLED history is most appropriate to assess a patient's past medical history.

3. Open-ended questions will provide the Paramedic with the most information.

4. You could speak to the patient through a family member who knows sign language or could write notes to the patient to assure adequate communication. Of course, you could also take a course in sign language at your local community college to help you better communicate with those who are unable to hear.

Practice Questions
Multiple Choice

1. a
2. d
3. b

4. b
5. d

Fill in the Blank

OPQRST AS/PN

6. onset
7. provoke
8. quality
9. region, radiation, relief, recurrence
10. severity
11. timing
12. associated symptoms
13. pertinent negatives

AEIOU TIPS

14. alcohol
15. epilepsy
16. insulin
17. overdose

18. uremia
19. trauma
20. infection
21. psychiatric
22. stroke

HAPI-SOCS

23. history of pulmonary disease
24. activity at onset
25. pain on inspiration
26. infection symptoms
27. smoker
28. orthopnea
29. cough
30. sputum

Chapter 16

Case Study

1. Decubitus ulcers is another name for pressure ulcers.

2. These ulcers are dangerous because they can become a source of infection.

3. You should use body substance isolation when in contact with patients with decubitus ulcers.

4. Pressure ulcers are caused by continued pressure supplied on one part of the body.

5. Pressure ulcers can be prevented by regularly turning the patient to limit pressure on certain parts of the body.

6. There are various answers the student may provide, but they may include: jaundice = decreased kidney function; cyanosis = hypoxemia; pallor = shock, and so on.

Practice Questions

Multiple Choice

1. b
2. c
3. d

4. b
5. a

Matching

Terms

6. r
7. l
8. i
9. n
10. t
11. b
12. g
13. m
14. a
15. h
16. j
17. e
18. q

19. f
20. o
21. k
22. d
23. c
24. p
25. s

Lung Sounds

26. d
27. b
28. e
29. c
30. a

Chapter 17

Case Study

1. Yes, there are occasions when splinting can do more harm than good.

2. This situation is an example of good clinical decision making. Although a novice Paramedic might resort to applying protocol-driven care in every situation, the experienced Paramedic can use clinical judgment to do the best thing for the patient.

3. You most likely learned from Wanda that experience sometimes teaches you more than protocols.

4. This answer will depend on the student's personal response, but most likely the answer will be yes. Students would be lucky to find someone like Wanda.

Practice Questions

Short Answer

1. The out-of-hospital environment is different from any other because of the spectrum of patient care that goes from life-threatening to routine. It requires synthesizing a great deal of information, and often requires the Paramedic to work under immense pressure.

2. Protocols and other guidelines only address classic patient presentations. They do not speak to patients with multiple disease etiologies, and they promote "cookbook medicine."

3. The components of critical thinking are concept formation, data formation, application of principle, evaluation, and reflection on action.

4. A Paramedic develops medical intelligence through medical knowledge, past experience, and use of a systematic approach.

5. A symptom complex is a collection of signs and symptoms.

Fill in the Blank

6. clinical
7. intelligence
8. syndrome
9. disorder
10. initial

11. Kaizen
12. protocols
13. check
14. mechanism, nature
15. emergent, urgent

Matching

16. e
17. g
18. b
19. c
20. d

21. i
22. h
23. f
24. j
25. a

Chapter 18

Case Study

1. This answer will depend on the student's personal response, but it may include that you know there is one patient who appears to be breathing. Since Ellie is alert, you do not expect that there is an environmental emergency such as carbon monoxide poisoning.

2. This answer will depend on the student's personal response, but it should mention that the first responders give you an update on what is going on so you can better prepare for the response.

3. This answer will depend on the student's personal response, but it should mention that 9-1-1 permits easy access to the system and that communications from the scene to responding units help you to prepare for the call.

Practice Questions

Short Answer

1. The primary advantage of using plain English rather than 10-codes is clarity.

2. Electrical interference in ECG tracings is caused by 60 cycle interference.

3. One of the earliest public safety uses of radio was hearing weather reports by the USDA.

4. Satellite phones are useful during disaster situations because telephone wires may be down and cellular towers may be overwhelmed with traffic. Satellite phones are not dependent upon cell towers or landlines.

5. The first 9-1-1 call was made February 16, 1968, in Haleyville, Alabama, by Rankin Fite, Speaker of the House of Representatives.

Fill in the Blank

6. first
7. notification
8. Communications

9. 9-1-1
10. digital

Matching

11. n
12. j
13. m
14. b
15. h
16. c
17. l
18. a

19. e
20. d
21. g
22. f
23. o
24. i
25. k

Chapter 19

Case Study

1. Your patient care report will recall the details of the call. You just need to review the PCR.

2. The best defense is simply to tell the truth. Do not guess. If you do not remember something, do not rely on your memory. Instead, give your answers from the patient care report.

3. By the time a case gets to court, you may remember little about a particular call. The patient care report chronicles the call from your perspective.

4. The PCR also functions as a medical document, and provides important information about the call to physicians and other healthcare professionals.

Practice Questions
Multiple Choice

1. c
2. b
3. c

4. a
5. b

Fill in the Blank

6. pertinent
7. medical
8. legal

9. black
10. line

Matching

11. j
12. o
13. m
14. c
15. d
16. i
17. a
18. l

19. b
20. f
21. n
22. g
23. k
24. h
25. e

Chapter 20

Case Study

1. Pediatric patients are more susceptible to gastric distention than adults because they have smaller lung volumes.

2. You can avoid the chances of gastric distention developing by ventilating with smaller volumes of air, using only enough to make the chest rise.

3. In relation to adult patients, pediatric patients have a more pronounced occiput; smaller airway diameter; larger tongue, tonsils, and adenoids; more friable mucosa; floppier and posterior sloping epiglottis; larynx position more anterior and superior; vocal cords pinker and angled toward feet; airway smallest at level of cricoid cartilage; and a trachea angled anterior and shorter. They are also more susceptible to gastric distention.

4. The most likely pathway to death for children is respiratory failure.

Practice Questions

Fill in the Blank

1. mouth, nose
2. nasopharynx
3. sinuses
4. nose
5. mandible
6. pharynx, hypopharynx
7. arytenoids
8. thyroid
9. vestibule
10. vocal cords

Matching

11. k
12. o
13. a
14. g
15. e
16. n
17. i
18. h
19. j
20. d
21. l
22. f
23. b
24. m
25. c

Chapter 21

Case Study #1

1. Your first step should be to open the patient's airway with the head-tilt, chin-lift method and check for breathing.

2. The next step is to ventilate using a bag-valve-mask.

3. The next action is to reposition the patient's airway and attempt to ventilate again.

4. If the breaths did not go in, you should perform foreign body airway obstruction procedures.

5. The airway algorithm helps the Paramedic to follow a routine pattern that is both familiar and methodical. In fact, the algorithm becomes second nature to the Paramedic. Although it does not encompass every situation that may occur, the algorithm allows the Paramedic to determine when a situation is out of the ordinary, and to act accordingly.

Case Study #2

1. You should suspect that the problem is something besides drowning, since the child wasn't found in the water.

2. You should open the patient's airway and attempt to ventilate. If the breaths won't go in, reposition the airway and attempt again. If the breaths still will not go in, perform back blows and abdominal thrusts.

3. If your initial actions do not resolve the problem, reassess the patient beginning with airway, then breathing, and so on.

4. When faced with an unconscious, apneic child at poolside, the circumstances point to an expected condition.

Practice Questions
Multiple Choice

1. b
2. c
3. d
4. c
5. a

6. c
7. d
8. c
9. b
10. d

Short Answer

11. If an airway cannot be established, quickly troubleshoot by repositioning the patient's head, suctioning the airway, and treating for obstructed airway.

12. If a second attempt to open the airway is also unsuccessful, you must assume an obstruction. In this case, you should follow obstructed airway procedures.

13. To ensure your first intubation attempt is the best one, assure that you have all your equipment ready prior to attempting intubation. Position the patient correctly, position yourself, and control the lighting. In short, make sure you are ready to perform the task before you begin the intubation attempt.

14. The four actions that meet the National Association of EMS Physicians definition of an intubation attempt are: (1) insertion of the laryngoscope blade into the patient's mouth, (2) insertion of a tube through the patient's nares, (3) insertion of a rescue airway into the patient's mouth, and (4) insertion of rescue airway devices through the patient's neck.

15. Intubation should be confirmed by verifying tube position through auscultation and one additional method, including an esophageal detector device or a colorimetric end-tidal CO_2 detector.

16. The use of algorithms can greatly facilitate airway management. However, it is important to recognize that the algorithm is written for the majority of situations, and that clinical judgment must also be used.

17. Five situations that call for active airway or respiratory management are non-patent airway, inability to maintain patient's own airway, failure to oxygenate, failure to ventilate, and anticipated deterioration of patient's status.

18. A potential problem when presented with an unresponsive patient who is not in cardiac or respiratory arrest is hypoglycemia or narcotic overdose.

19. Several circumstances in which you would provide emergency transport include abnormal vital signs unresponsive to treatment, unmanageable airway, ischemic compromise of an extremity, complicated delivery, uncontrollable bleeding, cardiac arrest reversal with abnormal vital signs, or cardiac arrest without defibrillation.

20. If the initial airway actions don't allow breaths in, reposition the patient's airway and attempt to ventilate again. If the air still won't go in, assume an obstructed airway and treat accordingly.

21. To secure an endotracheal tube, mark the depth of the tube, secure it with tape or a commercial device, and consider the use of a cervical immobilization device to minimize tube movement.

22. Blind insertion airway devices do not require direct laryngoscopy and are likely to succeed in at least partially securing the airway.

23. If you are unable to ventilate a patient who is not intubated, you should suspect airway obstruction.

24. If you are unable to ventilate a patient who is intubated, you should suspect tube dislodgement and/or obstruction.

25. If your patient has an open airway, is protecting his own airway, and is adequately oxygenating, you should continue monitoring the ABCs for changes in condition and move on beyond the ABCs.

Chapter 22

Case Study

1. You can use an oropharyngeal airway to help maintain the airway.

2. Gastric distention can be decreased by using cricoid pressure and limiting ventilation to that which is necessary to make the patient's chest rise and fall.

3. This answer will depend on the student's personal response, but manikin practice, continuing education, and assuring that you practice good basic skills are all common answers.

Practice Questions

Fill in the Blank

1. airway
2. basic
3. oxygen
4. nitrogen
5. decrease
6. 400
7. 660
8. 3,450
9. liquid
10. regulator
11. liters
12. 50
13. 10
14. 100
15. gag reflex

Matching

16. j
17. h
18. c
19. a
20. g
21. f
22. d
23. e
24. b
25. i

Chapter 23

Case Study

1. There are a number of devices available to help secure the airway, but the endotracheal tube is the gold standard in airway management.

2. The endotracheal tube provides direct access to the patient's airway, and allows for intermittent positive pressure ventilation, tracheobronchial suctioning, and the delivery of medications.

3. For endotracheal intubation, you will need a laryngoscope handle and blades, appropriately sized endotracheal tubes, a 10 cc syringe, stylettes, tape, Magill forceps, a tube-securing device, an end-tidal CO_2 detector, a stethoscope, and so on.

4. To ensure correct placement, you must also use waveform or colorimetric end-tidal CO_2 detection or gastric bulb.

5. It is important to prepare in advance for each intubation attempt since each attempt has the potential to cause bruising, bleeding, and other harm to the patient. The best intubation attempt is the first attempt.

Practice Questions

Fill in the Blank

1. Murphy
2. dual, or double
3. less
4. malleable
5. vallecula

Matching

6. t	16. k
7. s	17. m
8. p	18. i
9. n	19. r
10. e	20. o
11. b	21. f
12. l	22. j
13. d	23. c
14. q	24. h
15. a	25. g

Chapter 24

Case Study

1. Yes, this patient is a candidate for RSI since he cannot control his airway.

2. Yes, this patient's condition and the distance to definitive care warrants aeromedical transport.

3. The nine P's of RSI are **P**reparation; **P**redict the degree of difficulty; **P**reoxygenate; **P**retreat; **P**ressure on the cricoid; **P**aralyze; **P**ass the tube; **P**osition and secure; and **P**ost-intubation care.

4. The components of post-intubation care are an NG or OG tube, a long-acting nondepolarizing neuromuscular blocker, and a long-acting sedative.

5. This answer will depend on the student's personal response, but may include that RSI gives the Paramedic the best opportunity for a successful intubation on a difficult patient.

Practice Questions

Short Answer

1. The two agents commonly used as adjuncts to emergency rapid sequence are lidocaine and atropine.

2. In paralyzing the patient, the Paramedic takes full responsibility for the consequences of removing the patient's limited ability to protect his own airway.

3. Two tools used to perform an airway evaluation before and during airway management are the LEMON law and the 3-3-2 rule.

4. Administration of high-flow oxygen for three to five minutes or 10 to 22 deep breaths essentially removes nitrogen from the patient's lungs and replaces it with oxygen, helping to prevent hypoxia. This is why preoxygenation is important.

5. After the intubation tube is secured, place a nasogastric or orogastric tube, administer a long-acting nondepolarizing neuromuscular blocker, administer a long-acting sedative, and monitor with waveform capnography.

Matching

Rapid Sequence Intubation (RSI)

6. d
7. h
8. f
9. a
10. g
11. c
12. b
13. i
14. e

Pharmacological Intubation Adjuncts

15. g
16. j
17. i
18. f
19. h
20. a
21. b
22. k
23. d
24. e
25. c

Chapter 25

Case Study

1. Although you should consider the patient's history of "passing out," you should also take into account the bias of the patient's supervisor.

2. Although it might be easy to dismiss this patient's condition, you should keep an open mind and assess her objectively.

3. Some possible causes of hyperventilation include trying to blow off excessive CO_2, hypoxemia, inhalation of certain toxins, hormones, and so on.

4. Knowledge of acid–base imbalances can help you to better treat your patient by understanding what is happening physiologically.

5. An understanding of acid–base balance helps the Paramedic to develop clinical judgment. Clinical judgment is what sets a Paramedic apart as a healthcare professional, rather than a technician. If a Paramedic understands why the body responds in the way it does, she can better care for the patient.

Practice Questions

Multiple Choice

1. d
2. c
3. c
4. a
5. b
6. d
7. c
8. c
9. c
10. c

Fill in the Blank

11. hemoglobin
12. oxyhemoglobin
13. 20
14. acid
15. 0
16. 7
17. acidosis
18. alkalotic
19. oximetry
20. 95

Matching

21. f
22. b
23. e
24. a
25. h

26. j
27. c
28. d
29. g
30. i

Chapter 26
Case Study

1. You should ask the patient, "Are you allergic to anything, including latex?"

2. The parenteral route will provide the fastest effect.

3. The transdermal route is used for this medication.

4. Yes, the presence of the nitroglycerin patch might impact the amount of nitroglycerin you administer. You should find out when the patch was placed and how often he replaces it.

Practice Questions
Fill in the Blank

1. international
2. parenteral
3. enteral
4. buccal
5. Ewald

6. right, right, right, right
7. apothecary
8. metric
9. concentration
10. rectum

Matching

11. f
12. k
13. o
14. n
15. g
16. b
17. h
18. j

19. d
20. c
21. i
22. m
23. e
24. l
25. a

Chapter 27
Case Study

1. Yes, this patient is a candidate for IO.

2. Common cardiac arrest medications you can give via the IO line include atropine, epinephrine, and amiodarone.

3. A disadvantage of IO use is it is difficult to give a rapid bolus of fluids.

4. Some risks of IO infusion include pain, higher risk of osteomyelitis, fat embolism, fracture, extravasation, and compartment syndrome.

Practice Questions

Multiple Choice

1. c
2. d
3. b
4. c
5. b
6. a
7. d
8. c
9. c
10. d

11. c
12. c
13. a
14. d
15. a
16. c
17. c
18. b
19. b
20. b

Short Answer

21. The single largest drawback to IO infusion is the inability to infuse a large bolus of fluids.

22. Depending on the manufacturer, the IO needle can be placed in the sternum, the tibia, the femur, or the humerus.

23. Infants and children have more difficulty tolerating a fluid overload because immature kidneys have more difficulty adjusting to the changing electrolytes and fluid osmolarity that occur with a massive fluid infusion.

24. Four pre-existing medical conditions that can contribute to increased fluid loss include diabetes insipidus, emphysema, hyperglycemia, and alcoholism.

25. Crystalloid solutions contain electrolytes, whereas colloids contain proteins.

26. When a hypotonic solution is infused, water is drawn into the cells.

27. A macrodrip or trauma set will infuse fluid faster than a microdrip set. Similarly, a short drip set will infuse faster than a longer one.

28. The advantage of using a larger bore IV catheter is rapid fluid infusion and a decreased chance of clotting.

29. The advantage of using a smaller bore IV catheter is a reduced risk of thrombophlebitis.

30. Some of the complications of IO access include risk of fat embolism, fracture, extravasation, and compartment syndrome.

Chapter 28

Case Study

1. Before transport, you need to verify the patient's identity, consent for transfusion, the patient's blood type, transfusion orders, Rh factor, and that the blood is the correct blood type. You should also verify the blood is correctly labeled, not expired, and that the unit number and the patient information match.

2. While assessing a patient before transport, you should check vital signs, including a temperature.

3. If the unit of blood empties during transport, clamp the blood set and open the line of normal saline to keep the vein open.

4. You should check the patient's temperature since fever is a sign of transfusion reaction.

Practice Questions

Multiple Choice

1. a
2. c
3. b
4. b
5. a

6. c
7. c
8. d
9. a
10. d

Short Answer

11. Allergic reactions can occur due to mast cell activation in the recipient's blood from the exposure to the donor's blood.

12. TACO occurs when the patient receives more volume of blood products than can be handled by the circulatory system.

13. Acute hemolytic reactions are often caused as a result of A-B-O incompatibility.

14. Red blood cells transport oxygen to the body.

15. White blood cells work as part of the immune system and help to fight infection.

Fill in the Blank

16. clotting
17. 1
18. recipient

19. 15
20. eight

Matching

21. c
22. a
23. e

24. d
25. b

Chapter 29

Case Study

1. No, it is not unusual. In fact, in many cases some of the medications elderly patients take treat the side effects of the other medications.

2. When taking a large number of medications (some of which may not be current), the patient may have a difficult time keeping track of her medications.

3. Taking too much or too little of a medication may cause side effects.

4. Healthcare professionals who prescribe medications should take into account all of the medications that the patient takes, and prescribe medications accordingly. This is also an opportunity for patient education and counseling.

Practice Questions

Fill in the Blank

1. 50
2. therapeutic
3. distribution
4. reservoirs
5. bioavailability

6. action
7. receptor
8. agonist
9. efficacy
10. antimetabolites

Matching

11. e
12. a
13. m
14. i
15. f
16. j
17. c
18. b

19. o
20. k
21. d
22. g
23. h
24. n
25. l

Chapter 30

Case Study

1. The patient appears to be unstable.

2. You would expect his blood pressure to be low.

3. Classes IA, IB, II, and III may be effective on ventricular dysrhythmias.

4. The answer about medications will vary by EMS system. Since the patient appears unstable, synchronized cardioversion may be indicated.

Practice Questions

Fill in the Blank

1. catecholamines
2. dysrhythmia
3. bronchoconstriction
4. potassium
5. fibrinogen

Matching

Terms

6. a
7. o
8. h
9. m
10. i
11. k
12. c
13. g
14. b
15. f
16. j
17. d
18. n
19. l
20. e

Drug Types

21. c
22. b
23. d
24. j
25. g
26. e
27. f
28. h
29. a
30. i

Chapter 31

Case Study

1. You should expect hypoglycemia to develop.

2. You should ask the patient's mother, "Do you know if she took her insulin today? Did she take more than her prescribed dose? Has she eaten more or less than normal?"

3. The appropriate pharmacological intervention is 50% dextrose in water (D50).

4. Your patient's glucose level may have been disturbed if she took too much insulin or didn't eat enough to balance the dose of insulin.

Practice Questions
Multiple Choice

1. a
2. c
3. a
4. c
5. b

6. b
7. c
8. c
9. d
10. c

Short Answer

11. Insulin is produced in the beta cells within the islets of Langerhans of the pancreas.

12. Today's bioengineered insulin is identical to human insulin rather than being produced from animals and rarely causes allergic reactions.

13. Diabetes is the leading cause of blindness.

14. Type 1 diabetes is characterized by a total loss of insulin production, making life-long subcutaneous injections of insulin necessary.

15. Ipecac works by irritating the stomach and arousing the vomiting centers in the brain.

Matching

16. o
17. n
18. h
19. m
20. k
21. a
22. c
23. l

24. e
25. i
26. b
27. g
28. d
29. f
30. j

Chapter 32

Case Study

1. The only two rhythms that are irregularly irregular are ventricular fibrillation and atrial fibrillation. Since a patient with VF will have no pulse, you suspect atrial fibrillation.

2. Since the patient appears asymptomatic, you would likely provide O_2 and support during transport.

3. If the patient was unstable, electrical or pharmacologic interventions may have been necessary.

Practice Questions
Multiple Choice

1. d
2. a
3. c
4. b
5. b
6. c
7. b
8. a
9. b
10. a
11. b
12. a
13. c
14. d
15. b

Fill in the Blank

16. myocardium
17. diastole
18. chordae tendinae
19. ejection fraction
20. sinoatrial

Matching

21. c
22. h
23. a
24. f
25. d
26. g
27. j
28. e
29. i
30. b

Chapter 33
Case Study

1. No, the patient is symptomatic and hypotensive, so she is not stable.

2. Yes, it is possible. Although rare, some adults have a resting heart rate that is very slow.

3. The patient's rhythm is a complete heart block.

4. With a complete heart block, the atria is firing and the ventricles are firing, but they are doing so independently of each other. This results in a slow ventricular rate and low cardiac output.

Practice Questions
Fill in the Blank

1. calibration
2. corneum
3. warmth
4. Modified chest lead 1, or MCL1
5. anterior

Matching

Terms

6. m
7. o
8. h
9. b
10. j
11. g
12. i
13. c
14. e
15. a
16. k
17. d
18. f
19. l
20. n

Cardiac Rhythm

21. d
22. b
23. e
24. c
25. a

Chapter 34

Case Study

1. An early 12-lead ECG is important because a baseline ECG will provide a basis for comparison for future ECGs.

2. A 12-lead ECG can help the Paramedic estimate the location of the coronary occlusion, ascertain the ventricular wall involved, and predict the coronary artery that is affected.

3. No, the pain sounds like pleuritic chest pain of some sort rather than cardiac pain.

4. By running through the protocols in your mind, you refresh yourself on the possible treatment modalities.

Practice Questions

Short Answer

1. The primary advantage of obtaining a 12-lead ECG in the field is the identification of myocardial injury and the rapid transportation of the patient to a definitive care center.

2. The first negative deflection represents the depolarization of the septum.

3. Inverted T waves represent myocardial ischemia.

4. One of the first ECG changes associated with hypothermia is a prolonged QT interval.

Fill in the Blank

5. inferior
6. V1, V2
7. anterior
8. anterolateral
9. circumflex
10. global anterior

Matching

Electrode Placement

11. j
12. d
13. f
14. b
15. a
16. c
17. g
18. h
19. i
20. e

Terms

21. h
22. d
23. g
24. f
25. i
26. c
27. j
28. a
29. b
30. e